ULTRASOUND

for Advanced Practitioners

in Pregnancy and Women's Health

Cydney Afriat Menihan, CNM, MSN, RDMS

Perinatal Productions
North Kingstown, Rhode Island

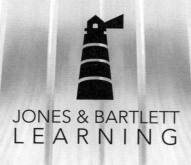

JONES & BARTLETT
LEARNING

World Headquarters
Jones & Bartlett Learning
5 Wall Street
Burlington, MA 01803
978-443-5000
info@jblearning.com
www.jblearning.com

Jones & Bartlett Learning books and products are available through most bookstores and online booksellers. To contact Jones & Bartlett Learning directly, call 800-832-0034, fax 978-443-8000, or visit our website, www.jblearning.com.

17172-3

Production Credits

VP, Product Management: Amanda Martin
Director of Product Management: Matthew Kane
Product Manager: Teresa Reilly
Product Specialist: Christina Freitas
Director of Production: Jenny L. Corriveau
Director, Relationship Management: Carolyn Rogers Pershouse
Project Manager: Lori Mortimer
Digital Project Specialist: Rachel Reyes
Product Fulfillment Manager: Wendy Kilborn

Marketing Communications Manager: Katie Hennessy
Production Services Manager: Colleen Lamy
Media Development Editor: Troy Liston
Rights & Media Specialist: John Rusk
Composition: S4Carlisle Publishing Services
Cover Design: Theresa Manley
Cover Image, Chapter Openers: © Deceptive Media/Getty Images
Printing and Binding: McNaughton & Gunn
Cover Printing: McNaughton & Gunn

Library of Congress Cataloging-in-Publication Data
Names: Menihan, Cydney Afriat, 1951- author.
Title: Ultrasound for advanced practitioners in pregnancy and women's health / Cydney Afriat Menihan.
Description: Burlington, MA : Jones & Bartlett Learning, [2020] | Includes bibliographical references and index.
Identifiers: LCCN 2018049425 | ISBN 9781284168457 (paperback)
Subjects: | MESH: Ultrasonography--nursing | Obstetric Nursing--methods | Point-of-Care Systems
Classification: LCC RG951 | NLM WY 157 | DDC 618.2/0231--dc23
LC record available at https://lccn.loc.gov/2018049425

6048

Printed in the United States of America
23 22 21 20 19   10 9 8 7 6 5 4 3 2 1

To Cecil Birtcher and his Birtcher Corporation, for hiring my dad and teaching him how to sell therapeutic ultrasound machines; and to my dad who practiced his ultrasound machine sales demo on me in our garage, thus planting the ultrasound seed. (1960)

To Dr. Rudy Sabbagha, who demonstrated the ultrasound machine to four University of Pittsburgh student nurses when no patients were in labor and there was nothing else to do. (1972)

To Linda Rondeau, first sonographer at Cedars-Sinai Medical Center Department of OB/GYN, who invited the nurses in to watch her do OB/GYN scans. (1973)

To an anonymous OB/GYN resident who launched my ultrasound clinical training when he said: "Watch me do this ultrasound and then you midwives can do them yourselves." (1982)

To Bob Adams, MD, and James Pretzer, MD, who taught me how to do ultrasound for ovarian follicle measurements and fetal gestational dating. (1984)

To Marshall Carpenter, MD, who asked me, "Aren't you a midwife . . . Who said you can do ultrasound exams?", sparking my quest for an answer to his question. (1990)

To the American Registry of Diagnostic Medical Sonography (ARDMS) which had the only answer, "Yes, we have a pathway for 'allied health professionals' to take the same OB/GYN certifying exam that sonographers take." (1992)

To the Association of Women's Health, Obstetric and Neonatal Nurses (AWHONN), which had the foresight to publish the first nursing guidelines to address nursing ultrasound practice. (1993)

To those leaders at the American College of Nurse-Midwives (ACNM), who listened to their members' concerns about incorporating ultrasound into practice, and convened a task force of midwife ultrasound experts. (2009)

To Lorrie Kaplan, former CEO of ACNM, who turned words into action. (2010)

To the American Institute of Ultrasound in Medicine (AIUM), which said, "We want to write joint ultrasound guidelines with midwives, but how do midwives demonstrate ultrasound competency?" (2010)

To Dale Cyr (ARDMS), for saying, "Sure, we can help you write an ultrasound exam for midwives" (2011); and to Tom Schipp, MD, RDMS, for jumping on board.

To all of the ARDMS staff who taught us the exam-writing process so it could be tailored to our scope of practice, now and in the future. (2016)

To those midwives who stepped up and took the first administration of the midwife sonography exam (2017); and to all those who follow . . .

To all of the ACNM and ARDMS ultrasound task force volunteers who unquestioningly gave their time, creativity, and expertise; and who charged forward with hot discussions and perseverance to further solidify the midwifery mantra "to provide safe passage to all mothers and babies" through education, training, quality care, and safe practice.

And finally, to Diana Dowdy, CNM, RDMS, DNP, and Kristen Ostrem, CNM, DNP, for trusting my judgment and supporting my professional quest, knowing it was filled with everything from bumps and divots to crevices and craters with but a thread for rope. I will forever admire your patience, thoughtfulness, and creativity, not to mention your inherent brilliance. I am in awe of your indefatigable dedication to quality pre- and post-graduate midwifery education.

– Cydney Afriat Menihan

2019

Brief Contents

Contents

Preface

Diagnostic ultrasound has become an indispensable part of nearly every clinical component of medicine and health care because of its accuracy, applicability, and availability, all of which continue to grow. The equipment is accessible in nearly all healthcare settings as some machines have become less expensive and pocket-sized. More providers are incorporating ultrasound into their scope of practice. Specifically, more and more nurse–midwives, physician assistants, and nurse practitioners are incorporating ultrasound into their practices as they become or continue to be the front line (or only) providers in office settings, clinics, urgent care centers, triage units, and emergency rooms.

When taking into to consideration all of the increases in availability and use cited above, it is no surprise that the number of ultrasound exams per pregnant woman is also increasing. From 1995 to 1997, the number of ultrasounds performed per pregnancy was 1.5. That increased to 2.7 ultrasounds per pregnant in 2005–2006 (Siddique, Lauderdale, VanderWeele, & Landos, 2009). This near doubling does not include the quick, unscheduled, unbilled ultrasounds performed to determine presenting part in labor, location of fetal heart, fluid checks, etc.

The overall number of nonphysician providers in general is also increasing (Corley, 2017). In 2016, there were 203,800 jobs in the United States for nurse anesthetists, nurse–midwives, and nurse practitioners. The U.S. Bureau of Labor Statistics (2016a) estimates this group will grow 30.4% (64,200 more jobs) between 2014 and 2024. In 2016, the number of physician assistants in the United States was 106,200, with the prediction it will rise 37% (39,600 more jobs) by 2026 (Bureau of Labor Statistics, 2016b; National Commission on Certification of Physician Assistants (NCCPA), 2016).

One conclusion easily surmised from these trending numbers is that the need for ultrasound didactic and clinical education is also increasing and will continue to increase for years to come. This fact leads to the unanswered question as to how this education will be integrated into the advanced practice educational programs that already exist. Because the application of ultrasound is so widespread in health care, ultrasound didactic and clinical courses must be specific to the area of medicine that is practiced, unlike most newer medical technology which may be taught to the general medical community (e.g., electronic record keeping). To accommodate this diversity in educational background, the approach chosen for this book was to use the scope of practice to define the ultrasound educational content. In utilizing this approach, it became clear that some nurse practitioners and physician assistants who work in obstetrics and women's health care have a scope of practice that overlaps with that of midwives and, therefore, could benefit from the same educational resources. Based on that premise, this book was designed with all of those advanced practitioners in mind.

For the purpose of this text, the term "advanced practitioners (AP)" will be used when referencing nonphysician providers such as family nurse practitioners (FNPs), OB/GYN nurse practitioners (NPs), nurses in reproductive health and urogynecology, nurse–midwives (CNMs), certified midwives (CMs), OB/GYN physician assistants (PAs), and any other healthcare provider with similar advanced education and training and scope of practice.

Finally, pertaining to the referencing in this book, the readers will note that some references are "old," the use of which is frowned upon. With all due respect, this author feels very strongly that credit should be given to those who planted the foundation for the technology that is still being used. If their measurements and graphs have proven the test of time, the nod goes to them rather than to a newer reference that retested their study and found it still to be true. In some cases, there just aren't any new references, which also says a lot.

Cydney Afriat Menihan

▶ References

Bureau of Labor Statistics, U.S. Department of Labor. (2016a). Occupational outlook handbook: Nurse anesthetists, nurse midwives, and nurse practitioners. Retrieved from http://www.bls.gov/ooh/healthcare/nurse-anesthetists-nurse-midwives-and-nurse-practitioners.htm

Bureau of Labor Statistics, U.S. Department of Labor. (2016b). Occupational outlook handbook: Physician assistants. Retrieved from http://www.bls.gov/ooh/healthcare//physician-assistants.htm

Corley, J. (2017, March 16). Advanced-practice providers are key to America's healthcare future. Retrieved from https:///www.forbes.com/sites/realspin/2017/03/16/advanced-practice-providers-are-key-to-americas-healthcare-future/#22b985645998

National Commission on Certification of Physician Assistants (NCCPA). (2016, March). 2015 statistical profile of certified physician assistants: An annual report of the National Commission on Certification on of Physician Assistants. Retrieved from http://www.nccpa.net/research

Siddique, J., Lauderdale, D. S., VanderWeele, T. J., & Landos, J. D. (2009). Trends in prenatal ultrasound use in the United States: 1995–2006. *Medical Care, 47,* 1129–1135.

Acknowledgments

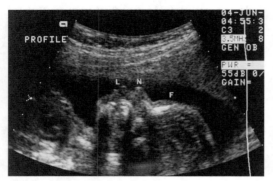

Courtesy of the author

The author wishes to extend heartfelt appreciation for the time and expertise generously offered by the contributors and reviewers. One set of eyes is never sufficient to ensure thorough coverage of the material and accuracy in its presentation. Also, a retroactive thank you is in order to prior contributors to other works in sonography that I edited: Judith Adams, RN, DN, DMU; Paula Cardillo, MS, RVT, RDMS; Sylvia Closson Ross, PhD, CNM; Marty Deviney, RT, RDMS; Diane Hodgman, CNM, MSN; Ann Holdredge, FNP, CNM, MSN; Carolyn Hopkins, BS, RNP, RDMS; Gale M. Kennedy, BS, RDMS, RT; Betty Kay Taylor, CNM, MSN, RDMS; Catharine M. Treanor, MS, RNC; and Wayne Persutte, BS, RDMS.

And a very special thank you for sharing images for this edition:
Betty Kay Taylor, CNM, MSN, RDMS
Diana Dowdy, CNM, RDMS, DNP

Reviewers

Jeanne Gottlieb, PhD, APRN, CNM
Assistant Professor
University of Southern Maine School of Nursing
Portland, ME

Linda A. Graf, DNP, CNM, WHNP-C, APN
Assistant Clinical Professor
DePaul University School of Nursing
Chicago, IL

Nicole Murn, DNP, CNM
Instructor (Clinical)
Wayne State University
Detroit, MI

Tammy Sadighi, DNP, ARNP, MBA
Assistant Professor
Florida Gulf Coast University
Fort Myers, FL

Donna Scemons, PhD, FNP-C, CNS
FNP Option Coordinator
Patricia A. Chin School of Nursing
California State University at Los Angeles
Los Angeles, CA

Maridee Shogren, DNP, CNM
Clinical Associate Professor, DNP Program
    Director
University of North Dakota
Grand Forks, ND

MaryAnn Troiano, DNP, APN-C
Associate Professor
Monmouth University
Middletown, NJ

Peggy Van Dyke, DNP, FNP-BC
Dean and Associate Professor
School of Nursing
Missouri Valley College
Sedalia, MO

Michael Villwock, MS, FNP-BC, CNM
Instructor, Course Designer
Simmons College
Boston, MA

CHAPTER 1

Ultrasound Guidelines, Education, and Professional Responsibility

▶ Introduction

During the past few decades, sonography has become an integral and vital tool in all aspects of health care, particularly during "point-of-care" (POC) applications. POC ultrasound examination allows for a quick and definitive evaluation to be performed when the patient presents with a complaint in almost any setting—for example, a medical office, an ambulance, the military field, a hospital emergency room, an urgent care center, and a clinic. Its reach is astonishingly broad and, in most cases, allows for rapid treatment. The adoption of such POC technology also supports the shift from the curative medicine of the past to the preemptive medicine of today (National Institutes of Health [NIH], 2010).

Sonography is now being offered as the first-line, "ultrasound first," assessment in the diagnosis and treatment of many healthcare issues (Minton & Abuhamad, 2013); the term *first line* indicates it is the medical imaging modality of choice in many

diagnostic situation due to its nonionizing radiation. Indeed, the application of sonography has become such an essential part of health care that use of this technology is now being taught in many medical schools throughout the United States beginning in the first year of medical school (Hoppmann et al., 2006). In turn, the implementation of sonographic assessment has become a critical skill not just for specialized physicians, "….but for nurses and all healthcare providers, including midwives, advanced nurse practitioners (APNs or NPs), and physician assistants (PAs), collectively known as advanced practitioners (APs). For the purposes of this text, the term *APs* refers specifically to nonphysician providers of pregnancy and women's health care, as those practitioners' scope of practice expands by demand and launches them into the world of sonography.

Specific to women's health care and pregnancy, sonography is the imaging modality of choice for the evaluation of many signs and symptoms of

1

potential complications, such as vaginal bleeding in all trimesters, locating intrauterine devices (IUDs), assessing for residual urine in the postpartum woman, and evaluating the endometrium in perimenopausal and postmenopausal women (**TABLE 1-1**). In many hospitals, many labor room nurses are expected to have the minimum sonographic skills necessary to determine fetal presentation during labor when a physician or midwife is unavailable.

The majority of sonographic exams performed by APs take place during a specific encounter where the information obtained by ultrasound will immediately benefit the patient. The benefits of this type of POC assessment–specific ultrasound has been described by the American Academy of Family Physicians (AAFP, 2018) as:

- Improving clinical outcomes
- Reducing failure and complication rates during procedures
- Rapidly narrowing differential diagnoses

- Shortening time to definitive treatment
- Lowering costs
- Reducing the use of ionizing radiation of computed tomography (CT) imaging
- Involving patients in their diagnosis at the bedside
- Enhancing the patient–provider experience
- Engendering confidence in the diagnosis
- Improving patient satisfaction.

Thus, POC ultrasound is practiced in a variety of settings, utilized by a diverse set of healthcare providers, and demonstrates tremendous benefits to quality and safety in patient care. However, in some clinical situations, scheduled serial ultrasound examinations are also indicated, as in fetal biophysical assessment, fetal growth assessment, and follicular growth assessment. These types of ultrasound exams all fall under the purview and scope of practice of many APs and will be described more fully throughout this text.

TABLE 1-1 Selected Indications for POC Ultrasound Examinations

Obstetric Ultrasound Examination	Gynecologic or Postpartum Ultrasound Examination	Reproductive Medicine Ultrasound Examination
First-trimester vaginal bleeding and/or abdominal pain with positive pregnancy test: Pregnancy location, +/– (presence/absence) of cardiac activity **No prenatal care and presents in labor or preterm labor:** Estimated fetal age (biometry), estimated fetal weight (biometry) fetal cardiac activity, fetal presentation, placental location, amniotic fluid volume (AFV), cervical length **Third-trimester complaint of decreased fetal movement:** Biophysical profile, AFV	**Unable to void postpartum:** Assessment of post-void residual urine **Cannot feel intrauterine device (IUD) string:** Identification and location of IUD **Perimenopausal bleeding:** Measurement of endometrial thickness **Scheduled well-woman office visit:** Measurement of endometrial thickness	**Ovarian stimulation:** Location and measurement of ovarian follicles **Embryo transfer:** Identification of uterine position **Positive pregnancy test following embryo transfer:** Identify location of the pregnancy

▶ Past and Present Barriers to APs Performing Ultrasound Examinations

Past Barriers

Ultrasound technology became a more commonly used assessment tool in all areas of medicine when the availability of mobile, easy-to-use devices began to crop up in emergency departments, triage units, outpatient settings, and other locations. At the same time, however, the majority of nonphysicians, predominently APs, encountered multiple barriers when it came to officially incorporating ultrasound into their practice. Some of the observed barriers were justifiable concerns, but overcoming those concerns became an obstacle given the limited resources available for their remedy. The major concern was the quality and accuracy of the scans performed, which potentially affected patient safety. Although the vast majority of physicians and APs obtained ultrasound education and training through continuing education programs, in-service education, supervised training, and formal courses, some were trained on the job by trainers/educators who were not skilled themselves, and still others were self-taught.

As these concerns grew and the obstacles became even more significant, they led to a reverse impact on quality of patient care. APs often found themselves in the position of knowing the patient would benefit from an ultrasound exam, yet being forbidden by institutional guidelines to perform such assessments, which caused delays in obtaining the necessary exams. Even today, some state laws prohibit APs from performing any sonography. A second obstacle has been in obtaining insurance reimbursement for the procedure. Reimbursement for the procedure performed outside of the radiology or other sanctioned locations was denied by most insurance companies and federal programs such as Medicaid. The third obstacle applied to American Institute of Ultrasound in Medicine (AIUM) accredited facilities. Until recently, all AIUM-accredited facilities were required to have all sonographers be credentialed, yet no credentialing exam was available for APs. In recent years, most of these barriers have eased as education, training, and certification have become available, and laws have changed. However, this is an ongoing process yet to be fully resolved.

Present Barriers

Changes began to occur in part when several professional organizations established minimal ultrasound educational and clinical criteria, such as the American College of Obstetricians and Gynecologists (ACOG, 2016), the American College of Nurse-Midwives (ACNM, 2018), and the Association of Women's Health, Obstetric, and Neonatal Nurses (AWHONN, 2016). These professional groups have published guidelines or position statements regarding the education and training of their members who wish to incorporate sonography into their clinical practice. Nevertheless, before incorporating sonography into clinical practice, it is important for the AP to investigate the individual state's nurse practice act or appropriate state laws to determine the feasibility of adding sonography to current advanced practice. Once this has been achieved, hospital policies and procedures may be developed to address the minimal educational content, methods for measuring clinical competency, and risk management concerns pertaining to the implementation of sonography into clinical practice.

▶ Professional Societies' Guidelines

Traditionally, the vast majority of obstetric and gynecologic sonograms have been performed by sonographers, radiologists, and physicians from other specialties who have incorporated ultrasound into their clinical practice. Professional organizations such as the American College of Radiology (ARC) and the AIUM have published guidelines that set general recommendations as to what should be included for each type of complete sonogram.

American Institute of Ultrasound in Medicine

AIUM is a multidisciplinary professional organization whose membership consists of physicians, APs, nurses, sonographers, and others from various medical specialties, with ultrasound practice being their common bond. Its primary goal is to promote the safe and effective use of ultrasound through education, research, guideline publications, and accreditation of facilities where ultrasound is performed. AIUM also works in conjunction with other medical and nursing specialties to develop joint clinical and practice guidelines that pertain to a specific type of practice. The AIUM Practice Parameter for the Performance of Standard Diagnostic Obstetric Ultrasound Exams, written in conjunction with ACOG, is an example of this kind of collaborative work (AIUM, 2018c).

AIUM Practice Guideline for the Performance of Obstetric Ultrasound Examinations

In 2013, AIUM revised its obstetric guidelines in conjunction and collaboration with ACOG, SMFM, ARC, and others. Personnel requirements and other aspects specific to the area of specialization (i.e., obstetrician versus radiologist) are addressed by the specific professional organizations. Additionally, the AIUM document stresses that fetal ultrasound should be performed only in response to a valid medical indication while utilizing the lowest possible exposure settings (AIUM, 2018c).

One of the major changes in this guidance from other publications was the recategorization of the various types of sonograms; the revised terms were then adopted by other professional organizations. These sonographic classifications include (1) the standard first-trimester ultrasound examination; (2) standard second-/third-trimester examinations (formerly referred to as the basic scan); (3) limited examination; and (4) specialized examination (formerly referred to as a comprehensive or targeted scan) (AIUM, 2018c). Because ACOG not only coauthored this guideline but also adopted this classification system for its own guideline, the details

for each classification will be provided later in this chapter along with other content from the ACOG (2016) obstetric guideline.

The AIUM guideline also provides information about the anatomic landmarks needed for each specific fetal measurement and serves as an excellent document for use in the clinical practicum. AIUM members have access to an online enhanced version of this guideline that shows images of each fetal anatomic landmark with proper cursor placement (AIUM, 2013a) for standard obstetric measurements.

AIUM Practice Guideline for the Performance of the Ultrasound Examination of the Female Pelvis

As with obstetric ultrasound, AIUM recommends that scanning of the female pelvis should be performed only when there is an indication or a valid medical reason for the procedure. These indications may include pelvic pain, menstrual disorders, postmenopausal bleeding, abnormal pelvic examination, localization of an IUD, and evaluation and monitoring of infertility treatments. The guideline provides a complete list of the indications, as well as a description of the specific landmarks for measurement and evaluation (AIUM, 2009).

AIUM Practice Guideline for the Performance of Ultrasonography in Reproductive Medicine

Ultrasound is an integral part of the evaluation and treatment of women with infertility issues. Whenever possible, AIUM recommends that a transvaginal approach be used for the evaluation of each organ and anatomic structure in the female pelvis. A comprehensive pelvic ultrasound examination should first be performed to rule out pelvic pathology prior to the initiation of treatment. If all necessary images cannot be obtained with the transvaginal approach, then a transabdominal scan should be done. Also, if there is any question of a pelvic mass, a transabdominal transducer can be used.

Under certain circumstances, a limited pelvic ultrasound may be performed for a specific indication. Examples of a limited pelvic ultrasound include a *folliculogram*, which is used to monitor ovarian stimulation and for other procedures in reproductive medicine, such as ultrasound-guided follicular puncture for egg retrieval with in vitro fertilization, as well as embryo transfer (AIUM, 2012a, in press). The AIUM practice guideline also makes recommendations as to appropriate documentation of this type of sonography. For example, when a limited folliculogram is performed, the following should be documented: (1) the number of ovarian follicles in each ovary and (2) endometrial thickness and endometrial morphologic appearance (AIUM, 2012a, in press).

AIUM Training Guidelines for Physicians Who Evaluate and Interpret Diagnostic Obstetric Examinations

For the non-radiology-trained physician, AIUM has published recommendations for the education and training of physicians who are evaluating and interpreting diagnostic ultrasound exams (AIUM, 2015a). In some clinical situations, a physician may be interpreting scans performed by APs, residents, or other providers. The key recommendations for those physicians interpreting ultrasound exams performed by other practitioners should call for:

- completion of an approved residency program, fellowship, or postgraduate training that includes the equivalent of at least 3 months of diagnostic ultrasound training in the area(s) they practice,
- under the supervision of a qualified physician(s) as defined by AIUM,
- during which the trainees will have evidence of being involved with the performance, evaluation, and interpretation of at least 300 sonograms as delineated by AIUM.

In the absence of formal fellowship or postgraduate residency or training, documentation of clinical experience could be acceptable providing the following can be demonstrated:

- Evidence of 100 American Medical Association Physician Recognition Award (AMA PRA) Category 1 Credits dedicated to diagnostic ultrasound in the area(s) the physician's practice.

- Evidence of being involved with the performance, evaluation, and interpretation of the images of at least 300 sonograms within the prior 36 months. It is expected that in most circumstances, these examinations will be performed under the supervision of a qualified physician(s).
- These sonograms should be in the specialty area(s) in which the physicians are practicing and are clearly delineated in the document.

To date, researchers have not been able to conclusively determine how many scans in each category a clinician needs to perform to be considered clinically competent (AIUM, 2018c). In turn, none of the professional organizations has set a specific number of sonograms necessary to demonstrate competency in POC sonography. However, AIUM has determined that at least 300 cases are needed to acquire sufficient experience and proficiency with sonography as a *diagnostic* modality and to gain a base understanding of normal and abnormal. For those physicians utilizing ultrasound in subspecialty applications, at least 500 cases are required by the AIUM.

As for annual competency maintenance, the AIUM recommends a minimum of 170 diagnostic obstetric and 170 diagnostic gynecologic ultrasound examinations to maintain physician skills. Thirty hours of continuing education specific to obstetrics/gynecology (OB/GYN) every 3 years is also recommended (AIUM, 2018c).

AIUM Practice Parameter for the Performance of Limited Obstetric Ultrasound Examinations by Advanced Clinical Providers; and Training Guidelines for Advanced Clinical Providers in Women's Health Performing and Interpreting Limited Obstetric Ultrasound

2018 was a pivotal year for APs who incorporate ultrasound examinations into their clinical practice. Two significant documents were published by AIUM, but most importantly, these documents were written by and endorsed by a multidisciplinary collaborative committee comprised of representative members of esteemed professional societies of physicians, nurse–midwives, NPs, and PAs. The full impact has yet to be recognized, but there is no doubt the impact on clinical practice will be significant.

The practice parameter reflects the minimum criteria for a limited obstetric ultrasound examination that falls within the APs' scope of practice (AIUM, 2018a). Of great significance is that this parameter recognizes APs may be performing the ultrasound exam as a POC examination or as serial examinations, thus broadening the scope of ultrasound practice. The document also addresses the ultrasound classifications, qualifications and responsibilities of the practitioner, specifications of each exam, safety, and documentation.

The training guidelines establish the minimal educational level for each type of AP and then builds onto that the minimal ultrasound training and educational components, as well as the necessary qualified physician team support for consultation and collaboration (AIUM, 2018b).

American Society for Reproductive Medicine

The American Society for Reproductive Medicine (ASRM) has also published guidelines for registered nurses (RNs) who have had specific training and supervision to perform ultrasound examinations in gynecologic and reproductive medicine. These guidelines do not stand alone; they are intended to be used in conjunction with other nursing guidelines, state laws, and institutional policy that address practice in these areas of nursing. A limited ultrasound examination in gynecology and reproductive medicine performed by nurses would include determining the number and size of developing follicles, measuring endometrial thickness and appearance, and confirming early pregnancy (AIUM/SRC, 2008, in press, 2017, in press).

American College of Obstetricians and Gynecologists

In 2009, ACOG, in conjunction with AIUM, published a technical and educational bulletin pertinent to sonography performed by obstetricians and gynecologists. This publication updated all components and parameters for the obstetric ultrasound examination and included the three categories of ultrasound examinations established by AIUM in 2007: (1) the limited examination, (2) the standard examination in all trimesters, and (3) the specialized examination. When the ACOG guideline was updated again in 2016, these categories were left intact (ACOG, 2016).

Limited Ultrasound Examination. A limited ultrasound examination is a less extensive examination that may be dictated by the clinical situation requiring investigation, which is pertinent to both POC and serial ultrasound examinations. Indications may include assessment of amniotic fluid, presence or absence of cardiac activity, confirmation of the fetal presenting part, interval growth, evaluation of the cervix, and placenta localization. The exam is not "limited" in terms of time, as measuring for interval growth can be time-consuming; instead, it is "limited" in its scope. Specifically, a limited scan for interval growth does not need to include any assessment other than biometric measurements for growth—providing a prior standard ultrasound examination has been completed. Limited sonography may be performed by sonographers or specially trained personnel. Of utmost importance is that a limited examination does not replace a standard examination.

Standard Ultrasound Examination. A standard ultrasound examination (formerly referred to as "basic," "complete," "formal," or "level 1" ultrasound) generally is performed by sonographers in the radiology or ultrasound department as a prescheduled, planned evaluation in all trimesters of pregnancy. The first-trimester standard sonogram may be performed by either the transabdominal or transvaginal approach. If a transabdominal examination is not definitive, a transvaginal or transperineal scan should be performed. Although this differs from the AIUM guideline, the intent is the same: If all parameters cannot be visualized with one approach, then the alternative approach should be utilized. Per ACOG, the parameters for a first-trimester ultrasound examination include the following:

- Evaluation of the uterus, cervix, and adnexal for the presence of a gestational sac
- Documentation of the presence, size, and location of uterine and adnexal masses, such as leiomyomas
- Assessment of the anterior and posterior cul-de-sac for presence or absence of fluid
- The location of the sac
- The presence or absence of cardiac activity
- Fetal number

Presence of a sac but the absence of a definite embryo or yolk sac may indicate a pseudogestational sac, which may be consistent with an ectopic pregnancy. Transvaginally, an embryo should be visible with a mean gestational sac diameter of greater or equal to 20 mm.

Fetal anatomy should be assessed according to gestational age. It should also be assessed in patients requesting individual risk assessment for aneuploidy. Nuchal translucency should be measured during a specific gestational age and interpreted in conjunction with serum biochemistry.

In the second and third trimesters, the standard obstetric sonogram includes the following elements:

- Evaluation of the uterus, adnexal structures, and cervix (when appropriate)
- Evaluation of presentation
- Amniotic fluid volume
- Cardiac activity, including abnormal heart rate or rhythm
- Fetal number; with multiple gestation, the exam includes chorionicity, amnionicity, fetal sizes, estimation of fluid volume, and fetal genitalia
- Placental location, appearance, and relationship to cervical os
- Fetal biometry for fetal gestational age and weight
- An anatomic survey

Each component of the anatomic survey has been specified by AIUM (2018c).

Specialized Ultrasound Examination. A specialized sonogram (formerly referred to as a comprehensive or targeted ultrasound) examination is recommended when a fetal anatomic abnormality is suspected on the basic scan or based on prior maternal obstetric history. The specialized sonogram generally is interpreted or performed by a perinatologist who is also a sonologist (i.e., an obstetrician with specialized training in sonography), who examines the suspicious anatomic feature or abnormality. Specialized ultrasound exams also include fetal Doppler studies, biophysical profiles, amniotic fluid assessment, fetal echocardiography, or additional biometric measurements.

Overlap among the ultrasound examination categories is inevitable. For instance, evaluation of amniotic fluid falls under all three categories. Also, more extensive studies, such as assessments of interval fetal growth, originally were included in the comprehensive category but now fall under the limited ultrasound category.

Overlap also is noted between the descriptors "limited" ultrasound and "point-of-care" ultrasound, although the meaning of the two terms is similar. Both are defined as an ultrasound exam that is performed to gain specific information warranted by the clinical symptoms at the time of evaluation (AIUM, 2018c).

Association of Women's Health, Obstetric, and Neonatal Nurses

In 1993, AWHONN issued a groundbreaking specific educational and competency guideline for RNs performing what was then termed *limited sonography*. The document described the basic training, educational content, clinical practicum, and competencies needed by experienced OB/GYN nurses who wish to perform limited sonography.

However, following AIUM's 2007 and ACOG's 2009 changes in terminology, "limited sonography" was no longer an accurate description for ultrasound exams performed by nurses. Since nurses were performing some components included in each of the new categories, AWHONN expanded its professional guideline first in 2010, and then again in 2017. The new guideline, *Ultrasound Examinations Performed by Nurses in Obstetric, Gynecologic, and Reproductive Medicine Settings: Clinical Competencies and Education Guide* (4th ed.) describes the appropriate clinical settings for nurses who perform ultrasound, as well as the recommended didactic component and clinical practice for all types of sonography. It specifically addresses RNs performing POC ultrasound (AWHONN, 2016).

The AWHONN didactic education recommendation is to include didactic content and instruction specific to the type of ultrasound the nurse will be performing (**BOX 1-1**). For example, the didactic focus would be on gynecologic ultrasound for the RN who is working in an infertility setting. There would be no need for such a specialized infertility nurse to learn, for example, the components of a biophysical profile.

The clinical application of ultrasound is a separate educational experience that is performed under the direct supervision of an experienced sonographer, nurse, or physician who is trained in sonography. The precise number of scans a nurse needs to perform to be considered competent cannot be quantified, since competency in ultrasound is an individual skill (AWHONN, 2016).

The educational competency and clinical practicum provide the basic skills needed for performing ultrasound. Evaluation of learning can be by written examination, verbal exercises, one-on-one tutorials, image reviews, or case studies. Knowledge of hospital protocols and procedures and the appropriate lines of communication should also be validated (AWHONN, 2016). Once the sonogram has been completed, the nurse documents the findings and reports them to the requesting provider.

American College of Nurse-Midwives

In 2018, the ACNM published a position statement indicating that it is within the scope of midwifery practice for midwives to incorporate obstetric and gynecologic sonography into clinical practice. However, when electing to perform ultrasound exams, midwives need to follow the Standards of Practice for Midwifery, which specifies the requirements for expanding midwifery practice beyond the core educational competence (ACNM, 2018). Midwives can obtain the necessary sonography education and skills through midwifery educational programs or on a continuing education basis (Box 1-1). Once this is accomplished, the midwife should be eligible for financial reimbursement for those ultrasound examinations performed. Additionally,

---

BOX 1-1 Recommended Didactic Education in Sonography for Advanced Practice Clinicians in the United States

Didactic content may be incorporated into educational program curriculum or obtained as a postgraduate added skill. The following is the minimum recommended educational content:

- Physics and instrumentation relevant to the type of exam to be performed (e.g., physics of ultrasound, proper use of machine and transducer selection, as low as reasonably achievable (ALARA) principle)
- Required elements and components as described by AIUM for the specific exam to be performed (e.g., imaging parameters for each trimester)
- Required anatomic landmarks defined by AIUM pertinent to the type of exam to be performed (e.g., landmarks for biometry)

- Indications for exam (e.g., indications for POC examination versus the standard examination)
- Clinical implications of normal and abnormal findings (e.g., documentation, communication, consultation)
- Ultrasound safety (e.g., output, frequency, length of exams)
- Components of a complete ultrasound report (e.g., orientation of image, documentation)
- Client education (e.g., explanation of procedure, communication of results)
- Additional didactic content specific to the type of sonograms to be performed (e.g., first trimester dating versus cervical length)

Specialized examinations are performed by clinicians with additional experience and expertise.

Adapted from ACNM, 2018; ACOG, 2016; AIUM, 2018c.

state regulations, licensing, and facility credentialing should be satisfied.

ACNM's position statement also directs midwives to the education and training guidelines established by AWHONN, ACOG, and AIUM. Clinical competency can be established during the clinical practicum under the supervision of an experienced sonographer or other professional competent in the specific type of ultrasound examination being performed. Like the other professional organizations, ACNM has not made any recommendations regarding a minimum number of clinical education hours or number of performed examinations due to individual learning needs; therefore, the determination of clinical competency is left to the discretion of the supervising sonographer.

According to ACNM's 2018 position statement, midwives need not be proficient in all aspects of ultrasound, but they may tailor education and training to the specific exams being performed. Once he or she obtains the necessary didactic education, the checklist system for determining clinical competence can be utilized and designed to fit the ultrasound skill to be achieved (see Appendix A, Sample Checklist for Documenting Clinical Proficiency). For example, if the midwifery clinical practice requires only the ability to perform biophysical profiles, the education and clinical training may be limited to the specific procedure. However, for those midwives who plan to become certified by the American Registry of Diagnostic Medical Sonographers (ARDMS), the midwife sonography exam tests knowledge and skill for all potential ultrasounds performed within the midwifery scope of practice. The ACNM's position statement delineates specific minimum didactic content that should be included regardless of the type of ultrasound to be performed for midwives performing any type of ultrasound exam.

Additionally, a system for consultation, collaboration, and referral for abnormal findings must be established and incorporated into midwifery guidelines. ACNM (2018) also recommends that any midwife who plans to perform fetal anatomic examinations should consider becoming fully credentialed in OB/GYN sonography by the ARDMS. Performing a full fetal anatomic survey requires a greater depth of knowledge, education, and training than POC ultrasound, so it requires credentialing

equivalent to that skill level. However, the vast majority of midwives will be performing POC imaging and not fetal anatomic surveys.

▶ Licensing of Professional Sonographers

Society for Diagnostic Medical Sonographers

The membership of the Society for Diagnostic Medical Sonographers (SDMS) consists primarily of sonographers and other allied health professionals who perform *diagnostic* ultrasound. SDMS issues guidelines and opinions on many aspects of sonography. Its major function is educational, as it holds local, regional, and national meetings providing ongoing continuing education. SDMS has advocated for national licensing rather than licensing on a state-by-state basis, but nevertheless supports licensing of sonographers (SDMS, 2018). Prior to 2009, individual states did not require licensing of sonographers. The first state to enact such a law was New Mexico, on April 6, 2009 (H.B. 498, 49th Leg. [N.M. 2009]). States now requiring state licensing for sonographers includes New Hampshire, New Mexico, North Dakota, and Oregon (SDMS, 2018).

▶ Professional Responsibilities

Scope of Practice

Prior to assuming responsibility for any level of ultrasound examination, it is imperative to know exactly how the incorporation of ultrasound into the individual AP's practice fits into professional practice standards, state laws, institutional credentialing, and practice parameters. The state laws governing the specific professional group, such as advanced-practice registered nurses (APRNs), midwives (CMs/CNMs), and PAs may vary in scope of practice for each group, with some restricting ultrasound practice to sonographers and physicians.

In some states, legal restrictions prevent non-physicians from reading or interpreting radiologic tests. POC ultrasound requires interpretation and potentially diagnosis during the procedure and at the time of the visit, unlike radiology ultrasounds, in which the images are later read by a radiologist and the results then communicated to the provider. The same applies to billing for ultrasounds performed by APs, with restrictions being imposed by such entities as the federal government (through Medicaid and Medicare), individual states, and insurance companies. Additionally, the place of employment may have restrictions or limitations for the APs performing ultrasound.

Obtaining Ultrasound Education and Training in Pregnancy and Women's Health

Historically, ultrasound education and training were initiated by the device sales/marketing/educational specialist employed by the manufacturer and then enhanced with continuing medical/nursing educational courses, online courses, and/or in-hospital training by someone with a radiology/ultrasound background.

These approaches alone are no longer considered to provide adequate education and training; instead, credentialing in ultrasound has become the expectation. Most radiologists learned ultrasound as part of their residency specialty programs. OB/GYNs as well as other physician specialties may learn it either during their residency programs (often from one resident to another or through a formal rotation in radiology imaging) and/or through continuing medical education (CME). APs may have learned ultrasound through on-the-job training and/or CME programs. Obtaining the necessary ultrasound education and clinical skills can be challenging for most healthcare providers, including physicians. As a result of the diversity in ultrasound education, professional societies have developed educational guidelines for those who are in clinical practice and need to incorporate ultrasound into that clinical practice so as to encourage quality, consistency, and competency. Those guidelines were discussed earlier in this chapter.

Until recently, ultrasound education had not been integrated into either professional graduate medical or nursing core curricula. Roadblocks to integrating ultrasound education into medical school curriculum and advanced practice programs are valid and substantial, focusing on financial considerations and time availability (Dinh et al., 2016). Nevertheless, in recent years, ultrasound education has become part of the core curriculum at numerous medical schools throughout the United States. The curricular design and integration vary, however, with some schools offering brief, targeted sessions and others having more formalized programs. Numerous institutions have designed curricula to span the duration of medical school, including both didactic and clinical skill courses (Tarique, Tang, Singh, Kulasegaram, & Ailon, 2018). In these programs, all medical students are exposed to ultrasound education not just in OB/GYN but in all areas of medicine, such as anesthesia, pediatrics, surgery, and general medicine, to name a few.

Medical School General Ultrasound Education

Most medical school educators now agree that ultrasound should be incorporated into the medical school curriculum, but there are minimal data to show which milestones should be attained through the four-year program. The milestones are competency-based developmental outcomes that can be demonstrated longitudinally throughout the four years. However, no consensus existed among medical school program directors as to the specifics of these milestones until 2016, when Dinh et al.'s first study was published. Ninety core clinical ultrasound milestones were identified by 34 U.S. medical schools, and those 90 milestones now need to be achieved by all students before graduation. It is hoped that other programs will use these milestones as a guidance for their own institutions or tailor them for a specific group of clinicians such as a CNMs, NPs, and PAs.

OB/GYN Residency Education Programs

As of this writing, most graduate physicians entering residency programs have not had ultrasound education during medical school and may find themselves in OB/GYN or other residency programs where ultrasound is fast becoming a mandatory skill. Even for those who have had some ultrasound education in medical school, ultrasound skills specific to the medical specialty will be needed as well. Although the need for this education is recognized, increasing educational demands and limited hours have impacted ultrasound education, and a diminishment of its extent has been noted over time.

AIUM recently convened a multiple-society task force to develop and publish a standardized consensus-based curriculum and competency assessment tools for the performance of basic OB/GYN exams to be used in residency programs (Abuhamad et al., 2018; Benacerraf et al., 2018). This is a groundbreaking and forward-thinking program.

Physician Assistant Programs

PA programs and graduates of those programs have been faced with the challenge of integrating ultrasound into POC clinical practice for many years. Integrating this technology into clinical practice after having already graduated from a program creates a postgraduate educational dilemma covering many areas—sources of the education and skill, the scope of practice, new curriculum development, and setting competency assessment, to name a few. The American Academy of Physician Assistants (2018) has published information about its position on PAs performing ultrasound, the programs that added ultrasound education to their curricula, and information relevant to ultrasound education for practicing PAs.

Women's Health Nurse Practitioner Programs

There is no doubt that the crusaders in the successful integration of ultrasound education into NP programs were the leadership at the University of Pennsylvania. Since approximately 2001, ultrasound education has been part of that program's curriculum. At this time, this mandatory course entitled "Fetal Evaluation" is part of the women's health nurse practitioner (WHNP) and midwifery programs, with one credit unit being awarded for its completion. The course comprises 45 hours of didactic education and 9 hours of clinical experience (personal communication).

Family Nurse Practitioner Programs

Traditionally, family nurse practitioners (FNPs) have not needed to utilize ultrasound in their clinical practice, but that may be changing as family physicians have begun to incorporate bedside ultrasound into their practices and are in the midst of discussing adding it to the family medicine residency curricula (Flick, 2016). Spurgeon (2017) studied the feasibility of adding ultrasound didactic and clinical education to FNP programs. FNPs who work in the emergency department are finding a need for this skill, as are those providing any obstetric or gynecologic services. Examples of areas for application of bedside or office-based POC ultrasound include cardiopulmonary limited ultrasound exam (CLUE), vascular extremity examination for thrombosis, and abdominal examinations (Spurgeon, 2017).

Midwifery Educational Programs

Few midwifery graduate programs in the United States offer sonography education as a mandatory part of their program. One example of a program that has incorporated a formal ultrasound component is found at the University of California at San Francisco. According to the program leaders, it was added to their core curriculum in response to "growing student, alumni, employer, and community demand" (Shaw-Battista, Young-Lin, Bearman, Dau, & Vargas, 2015). Other programs offer electives in ultrasound education or offer it as additional training. Thus, the vast majority of midwives are likely to obtain their ultrasound education as part of continuing education.

In 2018, ACNM published an updated position paper for midwives performing ultrasound, supporting the implementation of ultrasound into clinical practice. This document references educational opportunities for postgraduate midwives as well as means to determine competency in sonography (ACNM, 2018).

Clinical Competency in Sonography

Obtaining clinical competency in obstetric sonography is a challenge experienced by most non-sonographers for several reasons. To achieve clinical competency in this area, one needs to be able to (1) perform scans under the supervision of a qualified and experienced person, (2) have access to pregnant women as models, yet (3) limit exposure time to the pregnant models (AIUM, 2016a, 2016b, 2017). The issue of performing the scans under appropriate supervision is becoming less of a challenge as more registered and professional sonographers are becoming available to provide this supervision. However, the issue of scanning live pregnant models has multiple concerns involving fetal safety. To address this, AIUM (2017) provides an excellent and comprehensive resource for educators who will be using live models for clinical practicum.

Implementation of Telemedicine in Ultrasound Education

Although there are currently many options within the United States for ultrasound didactic and clinical education, most require travel and expense. Many APs practice in more rural settings with limited resources and travel time to achieve the necessary education. Telemedicine and other technologies do provide a creative solution for some of these issues, as demonstrated in one small but creative educational program carried out in remote areas of Kenya (Vinayak, Sande, Nisenbaum, & Nolsoe, 2017), shown in **TABLE 1-2**.

Use of Simulators for Clinical Practicum

Due to these theoretical concerns for live models and their fetuses, alternatives to developing clinical competency using live pregnant or gynecologic models has led to the development of simulators. Some of these are currently being used through online programs, with other types of simulators being used in classroom or other settings. Multiple computer-based programs as well as pregnancy and gynecologic phantoms exist that can be used for clinical practice; they can be found by online searches.

Safety in Training and Research

Diagnostic ultrasound has been in use since the late 1950s. There are no confirmed adverse biological effects on patients resulting from this technology.

No hazard has been identified that would preclude the prudent and conservative use of diagnostic ultrasound in education and research. Additionally, evidence from normal diagnostic practice relevant to extended exposure times and altered exposure conditions is inconclusive. Even so, it is considered appropriate to recommend that when examinations are carried out for purposes of training or research, the subject should be informed of the anticipated exposure conditions and educated on how these compare with normal diagnostic practice (AIUM, 2016a, 2016b).

Guidelines for Hands-on Scanning in Pregnant Subjects for Clinical Education

AIUM (2017) has addressed the appropriate use of ultrasound in education, with emphasis on safety for pregnant human models, during AIUM-sponsored training sessions. Subject participation requires appropriate informed consent. The primary obstetrician providing prenatal care should be informed of patient participation. The subjects should be prescreened to attempt to avoid unexpected findings, but there also needs to be a plan to address unexpected findings should they be observed during the educational course. There should be no first-trimester examinations due to the theoretical risk of fetal exposure. Exposure time—that is, the duration of the "hands-on" teaching session—should not exceed 1 hour per subject in the second and third trimesters (AIUM, 2016a, 2016b).

In the situation where a prior screening ultrasound was not conducted before the teaching sessions, incidental findings in volunteer models have been reported in the literature. It should be decided in advance of any clinical practice how an incidental finding will be handled. Siegel-Richman and Kendall (2017) have developed a protocol for their facilitators to follow that can be adapted to individual programs.

Competency and Cost

The didactic course content for learning ultrasound has been clearly established (ACNM, 2018). It is

TABLE 1-2 Example of Midwife POC Ultrasound Training in a Rural Area of Kenya

Objectives:	1. Determine accuracy of images and reports 2. Evaluate performance 3. Implement teleradiology 4. Identify components of education 5. Determine needs for improvement
Rationale: 1. Extreme shortage of sonographers and physicians trained to perform ultrasound (both urban and rural) 2. Midwives can do ultrasound screening and identify high-risk pregnancy for referral	Training Protocol: Three self-selected midwives, each with less than 3 years of midwifery experience
	Didactic Education: 1. E-learning module with didactic component 2. Needed a 100% score to pass the written test 3. Could take the test five times
Tasks: 1. Identify midwives who want to learn 2. Compile and implement training curriculum 3. Establish ultrasound facilities 4. Transmit images 5. Have radiologist validate the report	Clinical Education: Training Period: 4 weeks with 1-hour lecture and 6 hours hands-on until direct observation Assessed for competency during the 6 hours as time progressed Exit exam given at the end, testing both written and practical skills The study investigator spent time with each midwife evaluating progress and skill

Results:
1. All three midwives passed the online e-learning module on the first or second attempt.
2. All three midwives passed their exit examination on their first attempt at the end of week 4.
3. During their training, the midwives completed 271 ultrasound exams that were analyzed by the radiologists.
4. Images were transmitted to the radiologists by the midwives using a cell phone, tablet, or modem.
5. Turnaround time was a maximum of 35 minutes from sending images to the radiologists to receiving validation of the imaging results.
6. Accuracy of the images and reports was determined to be 99.6%.
7. The midwives labeled 20 patients as being "high-risk" during their training time.

Adapted from Vinayak, S., Sande, J., Nisenbaum, H., & Nolsoe, C. P. (2017). Training midwives to perform basic obstetric point-of-care ultrasound in rural areas using tablet platform and mobile phone transmission technology: A WFUMB COE project. Ultrasound in Medicine and Biology, 43(10), 2125–2132.

recommended that midwives utilize the guidelines established by both ACOG (2016) and AIUM (2018c). Acquiring the clinical skills is a more daunting task since clinical sites are limited. In a study of family medicine residents, Dresang et al. (2004) found that clinical competency in performing fetal biometry and fetal anatomic surveys was achieved within 25 to 50 supervised scans. Nevertheless, a minimum number of ultrasounds under supervision needed to achieve clinical competency has not been determined for nurses or midwives. Attaining clinical competence is learner dependent and unpredictable.

Whenever nurses and APs implement a new procedure into practice, the issue of training and cost needs to be addressed. A wide range of studies in the current literature have addressed both training and cost of achieving sonography competency in the United States (Abuhamad et al., 2018; Shaw-Battista, et al., 2015; Spurgeon, 2017). As previously mentioned, a program in which midwives in Kenya were trained to use ultrasound, although a very small study, provides a jumping-off point for those who need to be very creative, effective, and efficient (Vinayak et al., 2017); its findings may be applicable to APs practicing in rural areas of the United States (Table 1-2).

Specifically pertaining to training nurses, an older but excellent study addresses many financial aspects of such training at the University of Pennsylvania Medical Center and School of Nursing (Stringer, Miesnik, Brown, Menei, & Macones, 2003). It was determined that nurses were able to acquire competency in ultrasound examination at a reasonable cost. In this study, the nurses completed 12 hours of didactic education and a clinical practicum consisting of 6 to 9 hours and approximately 15 ultrasound examinations, resulting in a mean time of 7.5 hours of training. The cost per nurse in 2003 was $1037.55 (equivalent to $1381 in 2018 dollars) (Smart Asset, n.d.). This cost can be further reduced by utilizing home-study programs for the 12 hours of recommended (at the time of the study) didactic education as compared with paying lecturers to present the information on an individual basis (12 hours at $41.28) as in Stringer et al.'s study (2003), which would be 12 hours at $56.00 in 2018 (Smart Asset, n.d.).

Documentation and Retrieval

After an ultrasound examination has been completed, a record of the sonogram needs to become part of the maternal chart (ACNM, 2018; ACOG, 2016; AIUM, 2009, 2018c; AWHONN, 2016). The sonogram needs to be documented with appropriate still images or video, or secured in an archival system, in case the sonogram needs to be revaluated or compared at a later date. The permanent copy of the examination should be labeled, and the results should be documented in the patient's medical record. For instance, if an ultrasound examination is done in the emergency department, the indication for the ultrasound examination, along with the findings and plan of management, should be documented. After consultation and/or discussion with a provider, further studies may be indicated. If the patient is not compliant or unable to be compliant with follow-up appointments, a method for follow-up and documentation specific to this issue should be established by institutional procedures and protocols as well (ACOG, 2016; AIUM, 2018c, 2018).

Ultrasound for Nondiagnostic Purposes

The use of ultrasound for pure entertainment or psychosocial reasons is discouraged by many organizations, including the U.S. Food and Drug Administration (FDA, 2017, 2018) and AIUM (2012c). AIUM advocates for the responsible use of diagnostic ultrasound for medical benefits only. As stated in its document "Prudent Use in Obstetrics," AIUM (2012c) advocates:

> The responsible use of diagnostic ultrasound and strongly discourages the non-medical use of ultrasound for entertainment purposes. The use of ultrasound without a medical indication to view the fetus, obtain a picture of the fetus or determine the fetal gender is inappropriate and contrary to responsible medical practice. Ultrasound should be used by qualified health professionals to provide medical benefit to the patient.

When AIUM receives information that a practice, company, or individual is offering or promoting ultrasound for entertainment or nonmedical use, it first verifies the complaint, notifies the FDA, and then notifies the alleged offender that it has been reported to the FDA (AIUM, 2012b).

Keepsake Fetal Imaging

In the past, hospitals or ultrasound practices had concerns about giving parents a keepsake hard copy of the fetal images. One of the negative fallouts of this stand was that "keepsake video imaging" companies began to spring up. For a fee, a two-dimensional (2-D) or three-dimensional (3-D) sonogram would be performed, and the parents could purchase videos, DVDs, or photographs of the fetus. The major concern associated with these easily available unregulated services is that any pregnant woman could have a nonmedically indicated sonogram in addition to her medically indicated sonogram(s), thus increasing the fetal ultrasound exposure time (FDA, 2017).

In response to this concern, AIUM published a statement recognizing that fetal sonography may have an impact on parental–fetal bonding (AIUM, 2012b); for this reason, parents may desire to have a sonogram performed to acquire a permanent copy of the images (AIUM 2016b, 2017). To support this belief and to diminish the number of nonmedically indicated sonograms, AIUM supports the following practices (2012b):

- Providing images or video clips to the parents during medically indicated ultrasound examinations
- Ensuring these sonograms are performed by appropriately trained and credentialed medical professionals (physicians, registered sonographers, or sonography registry candidates) who have received specialized training in fetal imaging

Consent for Ultrasound

The issue of obtaining written informed consent prior to performing a POC sonogram is still being debated. Often the circumstances requiring a POC ultrasound make it difficult to obtain written informed consent prior to performing the scan. Although whether written informed consent is needed may be an institution- or practice-dependent decision, it may be beneficial, at a minimum, to verbally inform the woman why the POC sonogram is being performed and which structures or organs are to be imaged. It may be of equal importance to add that the POC ultrasound is a specific exam being performed to assess a specific complaint and will not include all fetal structures or assessment for anomalies.

Liability Concerns Related to the Performance of Ultrasound

In this day and age, liability concerns hover over all healthcare team members. As more clinicians use ultrasound in their practice, there is the potential for the number of malpractice lawsuits to increase. The greatest concern is with inadequately trained personnel using sonography, leading to increased incidence of misdiagnoses and medical errors. In past years there have been anecdotal reports of clinicians performing sonograms for fetal presentation during labor and missing the presence of a twin, the absence of cardiac activity, or placenta previa. In one anecdotal report, a woman who had never had a radiology-performed ultrasound, but who had numerous biophysical profiles, had an emergency cesarean delivery for "fetal comprise," culminating in the birth of an undiagnosed anencephalic baby.

Shwayder (2017) presented an excellent review of areas of litigation in sonography. These areas include inadequate education and training of the person who performed the scan, the performance of an inadequate or incomplete sonographic exam, images that lack sufficient quality to make a correct diagnosis, inadequate supervision of the "sonographer," and inadequate maintenance of the sonographic equipment. In an effort to limit or prevent any of these issues from occurring, professional organizations have published guidelines that address sonographers' education and training, the parameters of a complete or a limited study, supervision requirements, and equipment maintenance.

Without a doubt, errors have also led to litigation (Bedigian, 2017; Shwayder, 2017). Shwayder (2017) notes that the types of errors that occur may include so-called perception errors—that is, an abnormality is noted when images are retrospectively reviewed— and interpretation errors—that is, an abnormality is seen but inadequately or incorrectly described or diagnosed. Other areas of litigation include failing to recommend further studies or procedures based on findings, communication errors of ultrasound results, failure to perform an ultrasound exam, failure to store images, and failure to obtain informed consent (Shwayder, 2017).

One notable example of an ultrasound error involved inadequate maintenance of equipment; it led to a $78.5-million verdict when an obstetrician was unable to visualize fetal cardiac activity, declared the fetus dead, and ordered a radiology-performed ultrasound. No ultrasound technician was available at the hospital, so it took more than an hour for the second ultrasound to be performed, at which time cardiac activity was clearly visualized. An emergency cesarean section was performed, resulting in a live-born child who was depressed at birth and developed spastic quadriplegic cerebral palsy. The hospital records showed that the ultrasound machine used by the physician for the first scan had not had any maintenance or service in more than 10 years (Millburg, 2012).

A review of lawsuits related to POC emergency ultrasound by Stolz et al. in 2015 found that between 2008 and 2012 there were five malpractice cases involving emergency department physicians. All cases involved POC ultrasound examinations within the scope of emergency physician practice; each featured either a failure to perform an ultrasound study or a failure to perform a study in a timely manner. None involved a failure in ultrasound interpretation or an ultrasound misdiagnosis (Stolz et al., 2015).

Another review of closed claims involving midwives (McCool, Guidera, Griffinger, & Sacan, 2015) noted 162 litigation cases involving CNMs/CMs between 2002 and 2011. In this review, ultrasound was not noted in any of the seven major categories of liability risk for midwives. However, as more midwives incorporate ultrasound into their clinical practice, they will face the same risks as experienced by physicians as well as other APs.

▶ Ultrasound Practice Accreditation

Both free-standing and hospital-based ultrasound practice sites can become voluntarily accredited by AIUM (n.d.). Such accreditation is a peer-review process whereby the practice demonstrates that it meets or exceeds nationally recognized standards not only in the performance of ultrasound, but also in the interpretation of diagnostic ultrasound. It is believed that accreditation will improve safety and quality of ultrasound evaluations and interpretations (AIUM, n.d.).

▶ Practitioner Certification in Ultrasound Practice

American Registry of Diagnostic Medical Sonographers

The American Registry of Diagnostic Medical Sonographers (ARDMS) is an independent, nonprofit organization that was originally established to credential qualified sonographers. It was established in 1975 for the sole purpose of administering certification examinations in all specialties within the sonography community. The ARDMS credentials include the registered diagnostic medical sonographer (RDMS), the registered diagnostic cardiac sonographer (RDCS), and the registered vascular technologist (RVT). In addition, other certifications are now offered in several types of POC ultrasound, as well in midwifery ultrasound.

Until 2017, any AP wanting to obtain certification in obstetric and gynecologic ultrasound had to pass the same exam that sonographers take; this exam also covers the sonographic *diagnosing* of abnormalities and pathologic conditions. Because the imaging diagnosis of abnormalities and pathologic conditions is not within the scope of practice for midwives, in 2017 ARDMS launched the midwife sonography certification exam, which is specific to the scope of practice of midwives. The certification process involves two steps: (1) successful completion of a written, computerized exam plus (2) a practical exam that includes the submission to ARDMS of eight case-specific ultrasound examinations (ARDMS, 2017).

There are several benefits to successfully completing the certifying examination. It provides verification of competency in a skill level beyond core competencies. It also increases the practitioner's scope of practice and allows for more thorough, timely assessments, particularly in the triage unit. In addition, some insurance companies or federal programs will reimburse for ultrasound examinations only if they are performed by a certified or registered sonographer.

ARDMS has been working in conjunction with other professional organizations to develop competency examinations for those practitioners who perform specific types of ultrasound examinations but do not meet the requirements for becoming a registered diagnostic medical sonographer. Because of this rapidly changing area of competency/proficiency examination, refer to the ARDMS website (www .ardms.org) to determine testing availability for specific practitioners.

Ultrasound certification is not mandated as yet by any professional or national organization or entity; it is a voluntary certification process, although some institutions or states may mandate certification as a job requirement (AIUM 2015b). AIUM (2018b) supports the hiring of only credentialed sonographers.

It is believed that by testing for ultrasound competency and knowledge, ultrasound certification can alleviate some of the issues faced by APs, such as hospital credentialing and privileging, insurance reimbursement, state laws, and liability concerns. Based on this belief, ACNM joined forces with AR-DMS to develop and implement a certificate exam specific to midwife scope of practice. This exam was launched in 2017 and is available to all ACNM-certified midwives who meet certain prerequisites and requisites (ARDMS, 2017). At the same time, ACNM's ultrasound education task force moved forward in assessing existing ultrasound education courses for midwives, as well as developing its own (ACNM, 2018). Although it is not mandatory for midwifes to become certified in ultrasound, it was decided that a voluntary certificate in ultrasound competency may provide a better foundation to support the integration of ultrasound examinations with clinical assessment.

Other advanced practice clinicians are also in the process of exploring an ultrasound certification in their areas of specialty. Some prefer certifying within their own professional organization (Monti & Norman, 2017) or leaving certification to the employing institution.

▶ Summary

Although ACOG appears to stop short of recommending a standard scheduled ultrasound evaluation of all pregnant women (2016), the breadth of indications for ultrasound in pregnancy almost guarantees that every pregnant woman will have some level of ultrasound during her pregnancy.

Many nurses and APs working in obstetrics, gynecology, and assisted reproductive technologies are incorporating ultrasound skills into their everyday practice. Many clinical situations encountered on a daily basis require the ultrasound evaluation to complement the physical assessment being performed so as to provide efficient, quality care. Delay in obtaining a radiology scan increases the risk of a poor outcome as well as increases costs.

These same clinicians possess the ideal assessment skills required for obstetric and gynecologic triage. Knowledge and skill in sonography can serve to enhance the success of triage, expedite evaluation and diagnosis, decrease patient anxiety, and decrease waiting time.

Many medical schools have incorporated and mandated ultrasound education into their core curriculum (Dinh et al., 2016). Some AP programs have incorporated some level of ultrasound education into their programs, be it didactic lectures, clinical hands-on practice, or simulator scanning (Shaw-Battista et al., 2015). Over the past few years, barriers to the practice of ultrasound by APs have been reduced. Now, with an ultrasound certification process in place for midwives, barriers to hospital credentialing, insurance reimbursement, and independent ultrasound practice may be diminishing.

Sonography requires the acquisition of specific didactic information and the demonstration of clinical competence. Once the skills are acquired, continuing educational competence must go hand in hand with continued practice. A realistic concern expressed by radiologists is that untrained personnel will utilize ultrasound. Dr. Roy Filly predicted in 1988 that ultrasound would become the new stethoscope. He said, "As we look at the proliferation of ultrasound instruments in the hands of untrained physicians, we can only come to the unfortunate realization that diagnostic sonography truly is the next stethoscope: poorly utilized by many but understood by few"

(Abella, 2006). Only proper education and clinical training can prevent this undesired outcome from occurring. Today, nearly all OB/GYN nurses and APs have a pathway to attaining both educational and clinical competency in ultrasound, which should lay Dr. Filly's concerns to rest.

Study Questions

1. What is a sonologist?
   a. Any kind of radiologist
   b. An advanced sonographer
   c. A physician sonographer

2. According to ACOG's obstetric guidelines, under which circumstances should an ultrasound evaluation of a pregnancy be performed?
   a. Every pregnant woman should be offered at least one ultrasound during pregnancy, usually at 18 to 20 weeks' gestation.
   b. There should be a maternal or obstetric indication for ultrasound evaluation.
   c. The woman requests a scan.

3. What is a "limited" ultrasound examination?
   a. A less extensive examination that may be dictated by the clinical situation
   b. A specific exam of a suspicious area, such as with an anatomic defect
   c. An exam performed whenever time does not permit a standard exam

4. What does a point-of-care ultrasound examination entail in obstetrics?
   a. All of the components of a standard obstetric exam
   b. The same components as a targeted obstetric exam
   c. It is dictated by the clinical situation

5. What are some of the recommended methods of achieving clinical competency in obstetric ultrasound?
   a. Practice on all consenting obstetric patients coming in for point-of-care indications
   b. A combination of supervised live obstetric scanning and use of obstetric simulators
   c. Supervised live scanning of pregnant models in all trimesters if simulation is not available

6. When ultrasound is used as an adjunct to labor assessment to determine the presenting part during a point-of-care encounter with a woman at 37 weeks' gestation and a complaint of decreased fetal movement and contractions every 5 minutes, it is:
   a. necessary to document detailed ultrasound findings in the maternal record.
   b. acceptable to document only significant positive findings in the maternal record.
   c. not necessary to document that an ultrasound was performed because it is unlikely that the insurance companies will reimburse for a POC ultrasound.

7. Which factor(s) can contribute to litigation in ultrasound practice?
   a. Being untrained in ultrasound and not performing a POC scan
   b. An advanced clinician performing ultrasound without first attaining certification in ultrasound
   c. Choosing the incorrect transducer

8. The Food and Drug Administration recommends that pregnant women should limit ultrasound exams:
   a. by avoiding color-flow Doppler when having a "keepsake" video done.
   b. to indicated ultrasound exams only.
   c. by having only one exam at 28 weeks' gestation that includes a "keepsake" video.

9. A perception error noted in medical malpractice ultrasound litigation is:
   a. a fetal abnormality is visualized and recognized but there is a failure to notify the provider.
   b. a fetal abnormality is visualized but misreported as another structure.
   c. a fetal abnormality is not detected at the time of the ultrasound exam, but the abnormality is visualized when the images are reexamined retrospectively.

10. When a POC ultrasound is performed, at a minimum, the patient should be informed that:
    a. a POC scan is as thorough as a scheduled ultrasound done in the radiology department.
    b. this scan is limited to the specific area to be examined and a more detailed scan may be needed at a later date.
    c. this scan is limited and a written consent delineating the limitations should be explained and signed.

References

Abella, H. A. (2006, December 1). Luminaries make pledge to recapture "lost" sonography. Retrieved from http://www.diagnosticimaging.com/ultrasound/luminaries-make-pledge-recapture-lost-sonography

Abuhamad, A., Minton, K., Benson, C., Chudleigh, T., Crites, L., Doubilet, P., . . . Benacerraf, B. (2018). Obstetric and gynecologic ultrasound curriculum and competency assessment in residency training programs: Consensus report. *Journal of Ultrasound in Medicine, 37,* 19–50.

American Academy of Family Physicians (AAFP). (2018). Point of care ultrasound. Retrieved from https://www.aafp.org/dam/AAFP/documents/medical_education_residency/program_directors/Reprint290D_POCUS.pdf

American Academy of Physician Assistants. (2018). Integrating ultrasound into PA practice. Retrieved from https://www.aapa.org/career-central/become-a-pa/integrating-ultrasound-pa-practice

American College of Nurse-Midwives (ACNM). (2018). *Position statement: Midwives' performance of ultrasound in clinical practice.* Washington, DC: Author.

American College of Obstetricians and Gynecologists (ACOG). (2016). *Ultrasonography in pregnancy: Practice bulletin.* Washington, DC: Author.

American Institute of Ultrasound in Medicine (AIUM). (in press). Practice parameter for the performance of a focused reproductive endocrinology and female infertility scan. Laurel, MD: Author.

American Institute of Ultrasound in Medicine (AIUM). (2009). *AIUM practice guideline for the performance of pelvic ultrasound examinations.* Laurel, MD: Author.

American Institute of Ultrasound in Medicine (AIUM). (in press). *AIUM practice guideline for the performance of a focused reproductive endocrinology and infertility scan.* Laurel, MD: Author.

American Institute of Ultrasound in Medicine (AIUM). (2012b). Keepsake fetal imaging. Retrieved from https://www.aium.org/officialStatements/31

American Institute of Ultrasound in Medicine (AIUM). (2012c, April 1). Prudent use and clinical safety. Retrieved from https://www.aium.org/officialStatements/34

American Institute of Ultrasound in Medicine (AIUM). (2015a, October 21). Training guidelines for physicians who evaluate and interpret diagnostic obstetrical ultrasound examinations. Retrieved from https://www.aium.org/officialStatements/59

American Institute of Ultrasound in Medicine (AIUM). (2015b, March 25). Employment of credentialed sonographers. Retrieved from http://www.aium.org/officialStatements/32

American Institute of Ultrasound in Medicine (AIUM). (2016a). Live scanning for educational purposes. Retrieved from https://www.aium.org/officialStatements/66

American Institute of Ultrasound in Medicine (AIUM). (2016b). Guideline for hands-on scanning of pregnant subjects in AIUM-sponsored educational programs. Retrieved from https://www.aium.org/officialStatements/30

American Institute of Ultrasound in Medicine (AIUM). (2017). *AIUM practice parameter for ultrasound examinations in reproductive medicine and infertility.* Laurel, MD: Author. Retrieved from https://www.aium.org/resources/guidelines/reproductiveMed.pdf

American Institute of Ultrasound in Medicine (AIUM). (2018a). *AIUM practice parameter for the performance of limited obstetric ultrasound examinations by advanced clinical providers.* Laurel, MD: Author. Retrieved from https://www.aium.org/resources/guidelines/LimitedOB_Providers.pdf

American Institute of Ultrasound in Medicine (AIUM). (2018b). Training guidelines for advanced clinical providers in women's health performing and interpreting limited obstetric ultrasound. Retrieved from https://www.aium.org/resources/viewStatement.aspx?id=70

American Institute of Ultrasound in Medicine (AIUM) (2018). AIUM-ACR-ACOG-SMFM-DRU Practice parameter for the performance of standard diagnostic obstetric ultrasound exams. Retrieved from: https://www.aium.org/resources/guidelines/obstetric.pdf

American Institute of Ultrasound in Medicine. (n.d.). AIUM ultrasound practice accreditation. Retrieved from http://www.aium.org/accreditation/accreditation.aspx

American Registry of Diagnostic Medical Sonographers (ARDMS). (2017). Midwife sonography certificate. Retrieved from http://www.ardms.org/get-certified/midwifery/Pages/midwife.aspx

Association of Women's Health, Obstetric, and Neonatal Nurses (AWHONN). (2016). *Ultrasound examinations performed by nurses in obstetric, gynecologic, and reproductive medicine settings: Clinical competencies and education guide* (4th ed.). Washington, DC: Author.

Bedigian, B. (2017). Reason for ultrasound-related medical malpractice claims against OB/GYNs. Retrieved from https:///www.gilmanbedigian.com/reason-for-ultrasound-related-medical-malpractice-claims-against-ob-gyns

Benacerraf, B., Minton, K., Benson, C., Bromley, B., Coley, B., Doubilet, P., . . . Abuhamad, A. (2018). Proceedings: Beyond Ultrasound First Forum on improving the quality of ultrasound imaging in obstetrics and gynecology. *Journal of Ultrasound in Medicine, 37,* 7–18.

Dinh, V. A., Lakoff, D., Hess, J., Bahner, D., Hoppmann, R., Blaivas, M., . . . Khandelwal, S. (2016). Medical student core clinical ultrasound milestones. *Journal of Ultrasound in Medicine, 35,* 421–434.

Dresang, L. T., Rodney, W. M., & Dees, J. (2004). Teaching prenatal ultrasound to family medicine residents. *Family Medicine, 36*(2), 98–107.

Flick, D. (2016). Bedside ultrasound education in primary care. *Journal of Ultrasound in Medicine,* 35(7), 1369–1371.

Food and Drug Administration (FDA). (2017). Avoid fetal keepsake images, heartbeat monitors. Retrieved from https://www .fda.gov/ForConsumers/ConsumerUpdates/ucm095508.htm

Food and Drug Administration (FDA). (2018, May 2). Radiation-emitting products: Ultrasound imaging. Retrieved from https://www.fda.gov/Radiation-EmittingProducts /RadiationEmittingProductsandProcedures/MedicalImaging /ucm115357.htm

Hoppmann, R., Cook, T., Hunt, P., Fowler, S., Paulman, L., Wells, J., . . . Smith, S. (2006) Ultrasound in medical education: A vertical curriculum at the University of South Carolina School of Medicine. *Journal of the South Carolina Medical Association, 102,* 330–334.

McCool, W., Guidera, M., Griffinger, E., & Sacan, D. (2015). Closed case analysis of medical malpractice lawsuits involving midwives: Lessons learned regarding safe practices and the avoidance of litigation. *Journal of Midwifery and Women's Health, 60*(4), 437–444.

Millburg, S. (2012, May 11). $78.5 million verdict follows ultrasound error. Retrieved from http://www.radiologydaily.com/daily /obstetric-ultrasound/78.5-million-verdict-follows-ultrasound -error/

Minton, K., & Abuhamad, A. (2013). Ultrasound First Forum proceedings. *Journal of Ultrasound in Medicine, 32,* 555–566.

Monti, J., & Norman, F. (2017). *Guidelines for clinical ultrasound utilization in clinical practice.* San Antonio, TX: Society of Point-of-Care Ultrasound.

National Institutes of Health (NIH). (2010). Fact sheet: Point-of-care diagnostic testing. Retrieved from https://report.nih.gov /nihfactsheets/Pdfs/PointofCareDiagnosticTesting(NIBIB).pdf

Shaw-Battista, J., Young-Lin, N., Bearman, S., Dau, K., & Vargas, J. (2015). Interprofessional obstetric ultrasound education: Successful development of online learning modules; case-based seminars; and skills labs for registered and advanced practice nurses, midwives, physicians, and trainees. *Journal of Midwifery and Women's Health, 60,* 727–734.

Shwayder J. (2017, October 11). Liability in OB/GYN ultrasound. *Contemporary OB/GYN.* Retrieved from http://www .contemporaryobgyn.net/obstetrics/liability-obgyn-ultrasound

Siegel-Richman, Y., & Kendall, J. (2017). Incidental findings in student ultrasound models. *Journal of Ultrasound in Medicine, 36,* 1739–1743.

Smart Asset. (n.d.). Inflation calculator. Retrieved from https:// smartasset.com/investing/inflation-calculator#2IqvGwZLPN

Society for Diagnostic Medical Sonographers (SDMS). (2018). State licensure. Retrieved from https://www.sdms.org /advocacy/state-licensure

Spurgeon, J. M. (2017). Point of care ultrasound (POCUS) by the family nurse practitioner in the primary care setting capstone project. Retrieved from http://thescholarship.ecu .edu/handle/10342/6101

Stolz, L., O'Brien, K., Miller, M., Winters-Brown, N., Blaivas, M., & Adhikari, S. (2015). A review of lawsuits related to point-of-care emergency ultrasound applications. *Western Journal of Emergency Medicine, 16*(1), 1–4.

Stringer, M., Miesnik, S. R., Brown, L. P., Menei, L., & Macones, G. A. (2003). Limited obstetric ultrasound examinations: Competency and cost. *Journal of Obstetric, Gynecologic, & Neonatal Nursing, 32,* 307–312.

Tarique, U., Tang, B., Singh, M., Kulasegaram, M., & Ailon, J. (2018). Ultrasound curricula in undergraduate medical education. *Journal of Ultrasound in Medicine, 37,* 69–82.

Vinayak, S., Sande, J., Nisenbaum, H., & Nolsoe, C. P. (2017). Training midwives to perform basic obstetric point-of-care ultrasound in rural areas using tablet platform and mobile phone transmission technology: A WFUMB COE project. *Ultrasound in Medicine and Biology, 43*(10), 2125–2132.

CHAPTER 2
Image Acquisition

▶ Ultrasound Physics

Ultrasound is "sound" that is at a frequency above the range that can be heard by the human ear. Ultrasound is defined as an acoustic oscillation or sound wave with a frequency greater than 20,000 hertz (Hz) or 2 megahertz (MHz) (American Institute of Ultrasound in Medicine [AIUM], 2008). For diagnostic purposes, ultrasound energy is transmitted into the human body, with the returning echoes forming an image. The echoes created by the returning signals are referred to as *echogenic* (producing echoes), *hypoechogenic* (producing low levels of returning echoes), or *hyperechogenic* (producing high levels of returning echoes).

The transmission of ultrasound energy from one place to another is termed *propagation*. Thus, the speed at which ultrasound energy moves is its *propagation speed*. The actual propagation speed depends on the type of substance through which the energy is transmitted. Sound waves propagate through matter by causing the vibration of molecules; in turn, the stiffness, elasticity, and density of the matter (i.e., liquid, tissue, bone) that the molecules make up determine how fast the sound waves move. Generally speaking, the stiffer the matter, the higher the velocity of movement of the sound (sound propagation). For example, compared to water, bone is denser and will produce a greater vibration of molecules and a higher propagation speed.

The frequency of sound allows for the differentiation of ultrasound instruments into certain categories. Frequency is defined as the number of vibrations that occur per unit of time and expressed in MHz. The greater the number of vibrations that occur, the higher the frequency, and the greater the MHz; the lower the number of vibrations that occur, the lower the frequency, and the lower the MHz.

Frequency also affects how sound waves are transmitted: The higher the frequency, the shorter the sound wave (i.e., wavelength), and the better the resulting resolution or image acquisition. In addition, frequency determines the depth through which sound can penetrate structures, tissues, and organs. For example, with higher-frequency transducers, the image obtained will have higher resolution; however, the depth of imaging ability will be compromised and deeper structures may not be visualized. With lower transducer frequency, the wavelength is longer, allowing it to achieve greater depth of transmission. The downside of lower frequency is that the resolution is decreased.

The ultrasound transducer is the component that transmits and receives energy. It is responsible for converting electrical energy to mechanical energy within the ultrasonic frequency range as it sends the ultrasound signal through the body. It then converts the returning mechanical energy back into electrical energy, which is displayed as an image.

The piezoelectric element within the transducer converts energy from one form to another. This element is composed of ceramic material. When electrical voltage is supplied to the piezoelectric element, it causes vibration at the element's resonant (operating) frequency. This resonant frequency depends on the element's thickness: The thinner the element, the higher the resonant frequency of the transducer, and vice versa. Transducers are manufactured with different thicknesses of piezoelectric elements, with this factor determining the device's resonant or operating frequency.

▶ Sonography Display Modes

There are two display modes for the sound waves that are being returned to the machine: A-mode and B-mode. A-mode represents amplitude modulation, which is a single-dimension display consisting of a horizontal baseline. The baseline represents time or distance upward deflections that indicate the different acoustic interfaces.

Obstetric and gynecologic sonography display modes utilize B-mode, or brightness mode, meaning that each echo returned to the transducer provides a "brightness-modulated" display. B-scans are B-mode displays that provide a cross-section of objects in real time. In the early days of sonography, the B-mode machines provided only static or frozen images. Modern machines allow movement to be visualized; these scans are termed "real-time" scans.

M-mode is a graphic form of B-mode display in which a single dimension represents the motion of an object, such as cardiac activity. M-mode measures distance over time, allowing the calculation of fetal heart rate. M-mode is primarily used in fetal echocardiography.

The echoes returning from tissue and bone have different degrees of reflection that produce the shades of gray in the image seen on the monitor or in the film or print. The denser the tissue, the greater amount of returning echoes, and the whiter or brighter-appearing the image. Fluid-filled organs lack the necessary density to reflect echoes back to the transducer; the majority of the echoes pass right through them. Therefore, fluid appears black. Such structures are referred to as being anechoic (no echoes) or hypoechoic (low echoes).

▶ Doppler Ultrasound Transducer Operation

Two basic types of Doppler transducer operation are used in medical ultrasound: continuous-wave Doppler and pulsed-wave Doppler. Continuous-wave systems detect both the transmission and the reception of sound wave simultaneously. Both continuous- and pulsed-wave Doppler studies are used to detect the presence and direction of blood flow through vessels. The *Doppler shift* measures the difference in the frequency of the reflected sound compared to the frequency of the transmitted sound. It depends on the *insonating frequency*, the velocity of moving blood, and the angle between the sound beam and the direction of the moving blood. If the sound beam is perpendicular to the direction of blood flow, no Doppler shift will occur, so there will not be any display of flow in the vessel. The angle of the sound beam should be less than 60 degrees at all times to obtain the most accurate measurement.

Pulsed transducers, also known as pulse-echo ultrasound transducers, send short bursts of sound energy into the imaged area. Return echoes are produced by the different characteristics or densities of the material being studied.

Color Flow Doppler Ultrasound

Color flow Doppler is a form of pulsed-wave Doppler in which the energy of the returning echoes is displayed as an assigned color. By convention, echoes representing flow toward the transducer are seen as shades of red, and those representing flow away from the transducer are seen as shades of blue. Color Doppler ultrasound, also referred to as color flow ultrasound, is a technique for visualizing the direction or presence of motion (typically blood flow) within an image plane. The color display is superimposed on the B-mode image, thereby allowing simultaneous visualization of anatomy and flow dynamics.

Spectral Doppler Ultrasound

Spectral Doppler is a form of ultrasound image display in which the spectrum of flow velocities is represented graphically on the Y-axis and time is shown on the X-axis. Both pulsed-wave and continuous-wave Doppler results are displayed in this way.

Duplex Doppler Ultrasound

Duplex Doppler is an image display in which both spectral and color flow are used simultaneously. This facilitates accurate anatomic location of the blood flow under investigation.

▶ Transducers

The choice of which transducer to use depends on the depth of the structure being imaged. The higher the frequency of the transducer crystal, the less penetration it has, but the better the resolution, and vice versa.

All transducers have a palpable indicator ridge, button, or arrow that indicates the orientation. The indicator ridge on the transducer corresponds with the indicator on the monitor (upper left of the screen image, sometimes the manufacturer's corporate logo) so that the operator can determine which side of the body is being imaged.

Ultrasound images are typically displayed as mirror images. Thus, depending on the transducer orientation, when facing the monitor, the left side of the screen in the image is the patient's right in the transverse plane or the patient's head in the longitudinal plane. (Refer to the "Scan Planes" section for additional information.) The top of the screen is where the transducer is located on the body. It is recommended that the operator hold the ridge under the thumb so as to not confuse direction during scanning. If the monitor does not have an indicator mark, the left side of the screen typically corresponds to the side of transducer under the thumb (**FIGURE 2-1A**). Parts B–H of Figure 2-1 demonstrate the visual progression as the transducer receives the image and the appearance of the image to the operator.

Each transducer has an inherent frequency that is a function of its crystal composition and shape. Many of the newer probes offer several frequencies within one probe. The frequency of the probe is determined by the propagation speed of the transducer material and the thickness of the transducer element. Four probe shapes are used in obstetric imaging: linear, sector, curved linear, and intracavity or endovaginal transducer. These probes typically range in frequency from 2.5 MHz, which is 2.5 million cycles per second, to 10 MHz, which is 10 million cycles per second. Probe selection is based on imaging needs.

The display or shape of the screen varies depending on the type of transducer used. The sector transducer produces more of a wedge-type format, whereas linear transducers produce a rectangular format (**FIGURE 2-2**).

Frequencies for the transducers used in transabdominal OB/GYN imaging generally range from 3 to 6 MHz, whereas endovaginal transducers use higher frequencies, 5 to 10 MHz. Transducers are expensive, often costing more than $10,000 because of their specialized functions. The transducer is the most often and most easily damaged component of the machine. If a transducer is dropped, the piezoelectric elements or "crystals" can be broken.

The differences in transducers relate to the resolution of the images they produce and their ability to delineate various tissue densities. For instance, a fluid-filled bladder or an area of fresh blood will have no or minimal echoes (anechoic or hypoechoic) returned to the transducer, so the image displayed will be darker than the surrounding tissues. As blood begins to clot and become denser, more echoes will be returned to the transducer and will be displayed as different shades of gray. The denser the tissue or reflector, the whiter or brighter (hyperechoic) the image will be. A combination of

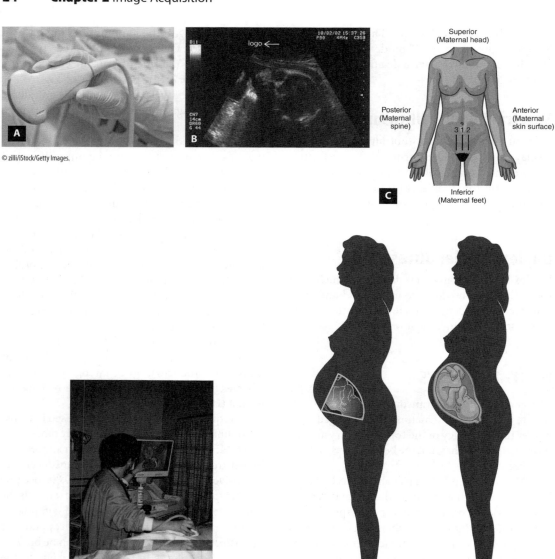

© zilli/iStock/Getty Images.

FIGURE 2-1 Visual progression as the transducer receives an image and it is transmitted to the operator. The notch on the transducer **(A)** corresponds to the side and/or the top of the monitor displaying the company's logo **(B)** to differentiate right from left and superior from inferior. In **(C)**, the notch of the transducer is directed toward the woman's head (superior). So, on the corresponding image (B), the top of the screen is toward the woman's head, the bottom of the screen is toward her feet, and the image is a mirror image of right/left (screen left is patient's right, and vice versa). **(D)** shows the relationship of the transducer placement (longitudinal) on the woman's uterus producing the image on the monitor. **(E)** takes that image off of the screen and places it on the silhouettes to show the ultrasound image in comparison with the fetal anatomic image. This example demonstrates how the fetal presentation can be determined by initially placing the transducer longitudinally, beginning suprapubically and moving superiorly toward the maternal sternum. The presenting part is under the transducer superpubically (vertex in the image above).

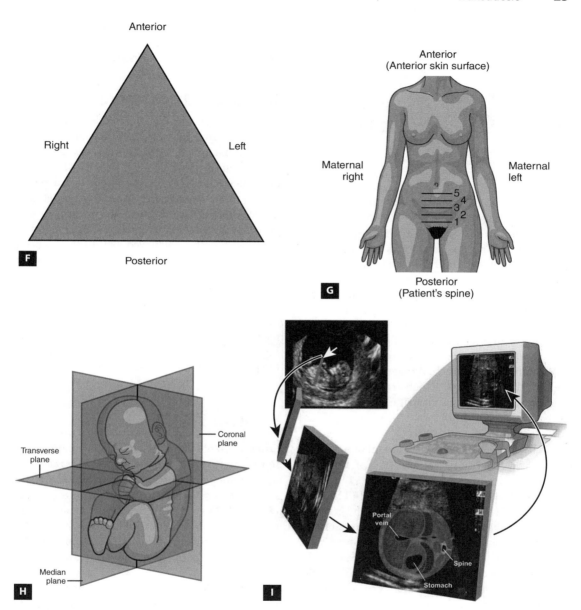

FIGURE 2-1 (*Continued*) **(F)** is a schematic representation of the monitor indicating direction and position if the notch on the transducer is positioned toward the patient's right side, in the transverse plane **(G)**. The top of the image corresponds to the patient's anterior, the bottom of the image is the patient's posterior, and the right and left correspond directly with the patient. **(H)** demonstrates the coronal, medial, and transverse (sagittal) planes of the fetus. **(I)** shows the progression of imaging from the time the transducer is placed on the fetus: First, a "slice" of anatomic structure is visualized by the transducer. That "slice" is then transmitted to the ultrasound monitor. In that process, the slice is "rotated" or "flipped" (similar to a slice of bread being removed from the loaf and "flipped" onto the monitor). Using this same type of demonstration, the fetal abdominal "slice" is taken and rotated prior to being viewed on the monitor.

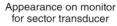

FIGURE 2-2 Monitor display formats for two types of ultrasound transducers.

fluid and tissue will appear in varying degrees of black, gray, or white.

An important concept to remember when choosing the appropriate transducer is that the higher the frequency of the transducer, the greater the resolution, but the shallower the penetration. Inversely, the lower the frequency, the lower the resolution, but the greater or deeper the penetration. The frequency of the transducer, the transducer diameter, and the distance/depth of the structure being examined are pivotal factors in the production of the image quality. Other factors that influence which transducer is the best option include the type of ultrasound exam to be performed. In obstetric ultrasound, these factors include the approach (abdominal versus vaginal), fetal gestational age, amount of maternal abdominal adipose tissue, and type of available transducers.

The development of transvaginal (TV) and endovaginal (EV) ultrasound has had the greatest impact on obstetric and gynecologic imaging in recent years, especially in the first trimester. Using the TV probe, fetal cardiac activity is identifiable as early as 4 weeks post conception, and ectopic pregnancies can be more accurately diagnosed. In the gynecologic evaluation, endometrial thickness can be easily measured with the TV probe. For the woman undergoing fertility treatment using advanced reproductive technologies, ovarian function and follicular response can be monitored and evaluated. Transvaginal imaging may even be implemented throughout pregnancy for those areas of interest that do not require deep penetration. These may include evaluation of the lower uterine segment and/or prior cesarean section scar, cervical length measurement, and evaluation of placental location in low-lying placentas or placenta previa.

Transducer Maintenance

Endovaginal transducers need to be cleaned and disinfected after use with each patient, following the manufacturer's instructions, which generally can be found in the product manual. There are different levels of disinfecting procedures, depending on probe use. AIUM also provides detailed instructions for cleaning and disinfecting the TV probes. When performed properly, a reduction in microbes be can be achieved, but it has also been noted that appropriate training in proper cleaning and disinfecting techniques has been insufficient. Multiple microbes, including human papilloma virus (HPV), have been identified on probes and probe covers. It is recommended that the probe itself also be cleaned by following protocols for high-level disinfection between each use should the probe cover fail (AIUM, 2018).

▶ Scan Planes

Orientation of the ultrasound image is paramount in the interpretation of the data. When referring to the scan plane, the terms most often used are *sagittal (longitudinal)*, *transverse*, and *coronal* (**FIGURE 2-3**). "Longitudinal" and "transverse" refer to the placement and relationship of the transducer to the anatomy (**FIGURES 2-4** and **2-5**). "Sagittal" and "coronal" refer to the view obtained by the probe.

The median plane is a vertical plane that divides the body into anterior and posterior segments through the midline of the body. The planes parallel to the midline are sagittal or longitudinal. At right angles to all of these planes are the coronal planes. The transverse plane divides the body into superior and inferior segments.

When the abdominal transducer is in the longitudinal plane, the "notch" indicator on the transducer should be pointing to the patient's head so that the

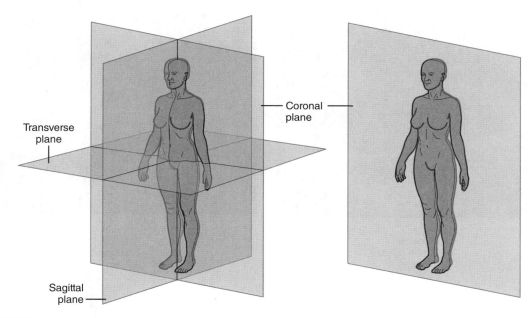

FIGURE 2-3 Anatomic plane terminology.

image on the screen presents the maternal head to the left of the screen and the maternal feet to the right of the screen. An easy way to check whether the probe is being held correctly is to place a finger under the transducer head and note which side of the image is affected on the display. Imaging in the transverse plane involves turning the transducer 90 degrees counterclockwise. In this plane, the patient's right is to the left of the display, and the maternal left is to the right of the display. This mirror-image approach (Figure 2-1) is also used for x-ray, computed tomography (CT), and magnetic resonance imaging (MRI). The instruction manual specific to the machine being used will describe the proper technique needed to acquire the appropriate image direction. In gynecologic imaging—as in all imaging—it is extremely important not to confuse the patient's right and left sides.

Coronal views divide the anatomy into front and back segments and are not typically used in transabdominal imaging of the female pelvis. However, the coronal view is used in transvaginal scanning and will be discussed later.

▶ Scanning Techniques

When determining fetal position transabdominally, begin with the probe in the longitudinal or transverse plane low in the pelvis or at the cervix, and then gradually move the transducer superiorly. The fetal part at the cervix is the presenting part. If the fetus is not in a cephalic presentation, follow the fetus's spine to the head. Next, find the stomach and the heart to ensure correct (left-sided) situs. This will determine the *fetal lie*. For example, ask yourself: Is the presenting part cephalic or breech? Is the spine toward the maternal left or right, anterior or posterior? Given this information, which side of the baby is up?

Transvaginal orientation of the image requires a different perspective. The scan planes are no longer longitudinal and transverse, but rather longitudinal and coronal. Transvaginal orientation takes practice to understand. Remember, the top of the display screen is where the probe is located, and the bottom of the screen is toward the patient's head (**FIGURES 2-6, 2-7**, and **2-8**).

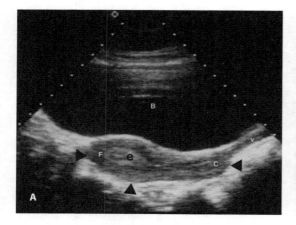

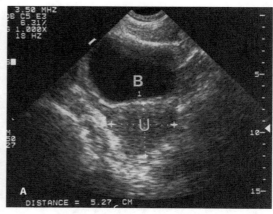

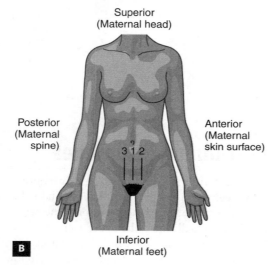

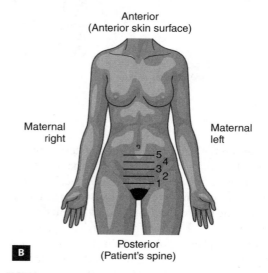

FIGURE 2-4 Transabdominal image **(A)** as seen on the display monitor with the longitudinal scan planes noted on the schematic **(B)**. The image demonstrates the maternal bladder (B) and the uterus (U) showing the relaxed detrusor muscle (DM) surrounding the inner mucosal layer (MU). In the longitudinal image, the body is divided into right and left, and the image is displayed as if you are looking in from the right side.

FIGURE 2-5 Transverse, transabdominal image **(A)** of a distended bladder superior to the uterus. Compare with the scan planes in schematic **(B)**.

▶ Abdominal Transducer Manipulation When Imaging

The movement of the transducer by the operator will greatly influence the quality and accuracy of the image. The following techniques can be used to improve the image acquisition:

- Slide the transducer across the abdomen to change the area of observation to a different slice or window.
- Use a window that minimizes the depth needed. This will increase resolution.
- Rock the transducer to focus on an area of interest or to broaden the field of view while staying in the same plane.

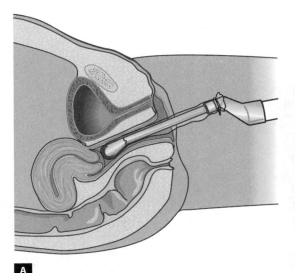

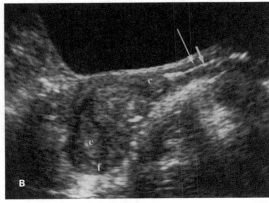

FIGURE 2-6 **(A)** Transvaginal probe and retroflexed uterus. **(B)** Transvaginal sagittal image showing the vagina at the large arrow. The small arrow indicates the white strip, which is the endovaginal canal.

- Rotate the transducer from the transverse to the sagittal to view the same structure but from a different angle.
- Compress the transducer against the patient's skin to improve contact between the transducer and the structure being assessed. Caution must be used with such compression as it can not only cause patient discomfort, but also alter the appearance and measurement of a structure, leading to inaccurate measurements.
- With obese patients, scan from the lateral approach, under the pannus or through the umbilicus, to decrease the depth needed.

Bahner et al. (2016) described prescriptive language that can be used when teaching transducer manipulation to new users so as to maximize the effectiveness of communication. This allows the learner to continue scanning without relinquishing the transducer to the instructor. Initially, scanning commences with "macro" movements to survey a large area. Then, the finer movements are used on the area(s) to be targeted by changing the angle of insonation, which is the angle of the beam to the organ or tissue of interest. Transducer manipulation changes the angle of insonation:

- Sliding: Transducer movement in the long axis across the body with a consistent 90 degrees to the area of interest.
- Rocking: Changing only the angle of insonation in the long axis with fixed body position.
- Sweep: Motion in the short axis of the probe with a consistent 90-degree angle of insonation.
- Fan: Motion in the short axis of the probe along a fixed point in the body and while changing the angle of insonation.
- Pressure/compression: Pressure on the probe, which compresses the body.
- Rotation: Clockwise or counterclockwise motion around the compression axis.

▶ Ultrasound Bioeffects: Thermal and Nonthermal

When ultrasound waves propagate or move through tissue, there is the potential for damage to that tissue. Theoretically, two known mechanisms can cause damage to the bone and tissue: thermal and nonthermal.

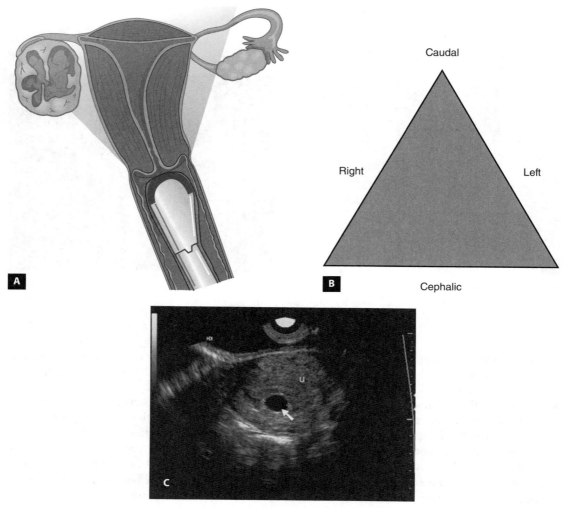

FIGURE 2-7 Transvaginal coronal view with **(A)** image and **(B)** schematic of image direction. The transducer tip (A) is at the cervix, and the transducer notch in this diagram is on the left. The cervix is closest to the transducer tip and represents the top of the monitor (B). The uterine fundus is farther from the tip of the transducer, so it appears at the bottom of the monitor screen **(C)**. The image is "inverted" in representation. Maternal right/left are the same as monitor right/left.

Thermal Effects

With thermal effects, the tissue absorbs the ultrasound wave and heat builds. Bone has the highest absorption of such energy, and its temperature can rise rapidly as a result. Adult bone absorbs nearly all of the ultrasound energy, whereas fetal bone heat absorption depends on the amount of calcification that has occurred. In soft tissues (i.e., organs), absorption is less than in bone. Water or amniotic fluid, by contrast, typically does not absorb ultrasonic energy and experiences little temperature rise.

The first potential mechanism for thermal effects depends on the volume of tissue exposed to the ultrasound beam. The greatest rise in temperature occurs in the area between where the ultrasound beam enters the tissue and the *focal zone*, which is where the resolution is the greatest. In addition,

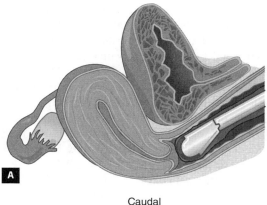

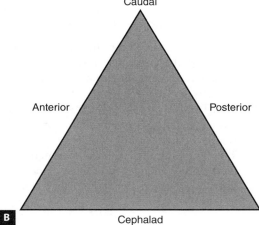

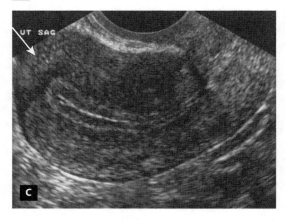

FIGURE 2-8 Transvaginal sagittal view. **(A)** Transvaginal probe tip at cervix. **(B)** Schematic of image direction when the transducer is in this position. **(C)** The acquired image from this transducer placement. The transducer tip **(A)** is at the cervix, and the transducer notch in this diagram is up. The uterine fundus is on the left (arrow), and the cervix on the right in **(C)**.

the volume of tissue exposed depends on the type of scanning technique: Is the beam moving or is it being held stationary? It takes time for the temperature to rise; therefore, the longer the transducer remains in one place, the greater the potential for the temperature to rise. Additionally, when ultrasound waves are transmitted in pulsed-wave form, there is a burst of energy and then a period during which no energy is transmitted. A cumulative effect may occur if the pulsed energy is used in a concentrated area over a prolonged period of time.

In scanned modes of ultrasound, such as B-mode and color flow Doppler, the energy is moving and being distributed over a large area. Therefore, the highest temperature is typically at the surface, where the ultrasound beam enters the body. For example, this is the case if the transducer is stationary and you are angling or heel-toeing the probe only.

In spectral Doppler, the power is concentrated along a single line, and energy is deposited along that stationary beam or *sample gate*. In these *unscanned modes*, the energy is focused over a smaller volume of tissue than is the case with the scanned modes, so the highest temperature is found between the surface and the focal zone. A good analogy for scanned versus unscanned modes is moving a hot iron over the entire piece of clothing versus holding a hot iron over a piece of cloth for a prolonged period of time; the heat is disbursed during the scanned time and concentrated during the unscanned period. Additionally, in an obese woman, the adipose tissue can absorb much of the heat; in contrast, in a woman with a thin abdominal wall, more energy is transmitted to the fetus. M-mode utilizes grayscale or B-mode scanning, so it does not increase the energy directed to the focal zone. For this reason, in the first trimester, only M-mode should be used to record fetal heart rate, not pulsed Doppler (AIUM, 2016a, 2016b).

The person performing the ultrasound examination has the ability to minimize the rise in temperature (AIUM 2014a, 2014b). Temperature increases depend on intensity, the duration of exposure in one location, the transducer focal point size and location, and the absorption of the energy. The intensity of the ultrasound wave depends on the equipment chosen for the exam and, therefore, is operator dependent. Likewise, the operator controls the duration of exposure. The fixed-focused transducers have a focus that cannot be changed, but the operator can change the focus on multi-element array transducers. Understanding how the equipment works is of paramount importance in reducing thermal exposure to the patient. The goal is to obtain the necessary medical images while using the lowest amount of energy and the least amount of exposure time.

Nonthermal Effects

Nonthermal bioeffects, also referred to as *mechanical bioeffects*, are not as well understood as thermal effects. They seem to be caused by ultrasound pressure waves passing through or near areas with gas or air pockets, thereby causing tissue motion. This phenomenon is known as *cavitation*. Cavitation is defined as the generation, growth, vibration, and possible collapse of microbubbles within the tissue. It is possible for cavitation to occur in diagnostic ultrasound, but there is no evidence thus far that diagnostic ultrasound exposure has caused cavitation in humans in the absence of gas bubbles. The main concern for creation of cavitation arises when contrast agents are used. To minimize the risk of cavitation, always keep the output as low as possible and keep the ultrasound examination time as short as possible to obtain the imaging information needed (AIUM, 2014a, 2014b).

▶ Output Display

The output display, which shows the indices that relate to the potential for bioeffects, is found on the image screen. These indices were established by the National Electrical Manufacturers Association, the U.S. Food and Drug Administration (FDA), the AIUM, and several other societies. The current standard is formally called the Standard for Real-Time Display of Thermal and Mechanical Acoustic Output Indices on Diagnostic Ultrasound Equipment, but more commonly called the Output Display Standard (ODS).

Two types of indices are displayed on the ODS: thermal mechanisms, referred to as the thermal index

(TI), and mechanical or nonthermal mechanisms, referred to as the mechanical index (MI). The goal of users of diagnostic medical imaging equipment is to acquire the best-quality images while keeping the TI and MI as low as reasonably possible (AIUM, 2014a, 2014b). An output display is not required if the equipment is not capable of exceeding an MI or a TI of 1. However, if the transducer and system are capable of exceeding a TI and/or MI of 1, then the display values must be displayed. Increments can be displayed as values as low as 0.4.

The thermal indices are only a relative indicator of temperature rise, not an indication of actual temperature. TIs are categorized into three types based on the density of fetal tissue being scanned:

- TIS: The soft tissue index indicates whether a change in the instrument setting will lead to an increase in temperature within soft homogeneous tissues.
- TIC: The TIC provides the same information for the cranial bone or any bone at or near the surface of the scanning plane.
- TIB: The bone TI provides information on temperature changes in bone at or near the focus after the beam has traversed the soft tissue.

▶ Ultrasound Safety: The ALARA Principle

The acronym ALARA stands for "as low as reasonably achievable." In ultrasound, the ALARA principle means that exposure should be kept as low as possible while still being able to acquire diagnostic images and needed information (AIUM, 2014a, 2014b). To accomplish this, when using ultrasound for any type of examination, always follow these principles:

- Use the lowest power to acquire the necessary image.
- Use the least amount of time to acquire the necessary image.
- Use power or color Doppler only as necessary.
- Do not use pulsed Doppler unless necessary because it creates the greatest energy.
- TI should be 1 or less.

▶ Image Processing

Transmission controls on the keyboard of the ultrasound machine allow the operator to control the ultrasound output and improve the quality of the image. The controls that affect the intensity are discussed next.

The *application selection* control allows the operator to select the type of ultrasound being done (i.e., fetal, ophthalmic, peripheral blood vessel). Different types of exams utilize different intensities. The maximum intensity for each type of exam is regulated by the FDA.

The *output intensity* control (also called transmit, power, or output) is automatically determined once the application or preset is chosen. However, most equipment allows the operator to change intensity levels.

The *choice of field for exam* control (i.e., B-mode, M-mode, or Doppler) is based on whether the ultrasound beam is stationary or in motion, which affects the energy absorbed by the tissue. If the beam is stationary, the targeted exam area receives increased amounts of ultrasound energy.

The *pulse repetition frequency (PRF)* control determines the output. The higher the PRF, the higher the output.

Focusing occurs when the beam is narrowed, which results in better lateral resolution. Improving lateral resolution means that the beam will be focused longer on one area. It is possible to set the transducer focus at the proper depth to improve the image of that structure without increasing the intensity.

Pulse length is the length of time the pulse is on. The longer it is on, the greater the likelihood of raising tissue temperature.

The *transducer type* control selects the frequency of the transducer. The higher the frequency of the transducer, the greater the output intensity needed to image structures located at greater depths. Therefore, if greater depth is needed, it is recommended to switch to a lower-frequency transducer to improve the quality of the image, so as to avoid increasing the intensity. Depth should always be adjusted to include the region of interest. For example, while performing a pregnancy scan, the operator can adjust the depth to include the posterior uterus, but there is no need to image back to the maternal spine.

Manufacturers are required to provide a default setting for the output levels that conform to safe levels. The default levels are automatically set when the machine is turned on but can be adjusted by the operator. If the output levels are changed, careful observation of the TI and MI is imperative. Also, if preset default output levels are being used, there is still a possibility of increasing risk of harm if the exposure time is not minimized.

A second set of controls, known as *receiver controls*, affect the image display without having any effect on the output. The receiver controls are controlled by the person performing the ultrasound.

- *Receiver gain* controls regulate the amplification of the returning signal or echo that is being reflected back by the tissue or fluid; they may be referred to as the *near gain* and *far gain* controls. When attempting to image a structure that is located deeper within the body cavity, increasing the far gain may improve the quality of the image. When imaging a structure located closer to the surface, increasing the near gain control may improve visualization of those structures.

- *Time-gain compensation (TGC)* or *overall gain compensation* is also known as the depth gain compensation (DGC). The TGC equalizes the differing intensities of received echoes, which may initially be unequal due to differences in reflector depth. For example, to visualize a fetal part that may be close to the anterior surface of the maternal abdomen and simultaneously visualize the placenta, which may be on the posterior wall of the uterus, the TGC would be adjusted so that the sound waves reflected from the placenta, which need to travel farther, are amplified and the sound waves being received from more anterior structures are dampened. This will equalize all of the received signals.

Many ultrasound machines come with an *automatic gain control* that will automatically adjust the gains to maximize the image quality.

Postprocessing of images includes such functions as the *cine-loop*. Cine-loop allows the operator to move backward or forward through the stored images to locate the best image frame for a particular measurement or for documentation purposes. Most ultrasound machines store multiple images while scanning; this allows the operator to "rewind" or look back through prior images to find the best view of the area of interest.

▶ Basic Controls and Settings

Overall gain does not change the frequency or the intensity of the transducer. Instead, it determines how much amplification is accomplished in the receiver of the transducer; it is similar to the volume control on a stereo system. Most of the work done by the transducer is done in the "listening" phase of the process. Less than 1% of the transducer's time is spent in transmitting sound waves into the body, leaving more than 99% of the time designated just for receiving the signals. This is called *duty cycle* or *duty factor*.

As noted earlier, the TGC equalizes the differing intensity of received echoes, which may initially be unequal due to differences in reflector depth. For example, when visualizing the posterior uterus in an obese patient, more ultrasound waves are absorbed. In this case, the TGC slope may be steeper than in a patient of normal habitus.

▶ Artifacts

Artifacts are distortions of the anatomic structures on the image. Proper adjustment of two operator-dependent variables—overall gain and TGC—along with appropriate transducer selection can eliminate many of the artifacts commonly seen in ultrasound imaging.

The application of coupling gel eliminates the most common imaging artifacts. Gel is a liquid medium that allows the ultrasound beam to be transmitted through the skin. Gel is also used with the transvaginal probes for the same purpose. The gel itself has the potential for transmitting pathogens and, therefore, an infection control policy regarding

the use of ultrasound coupling gel and appropriate training of staff is imperative (AIUM, 2018). Also, a steady contact between the transducer and the skin or body surface will eliminate air getting between the transducer and the skin, which will diminish or eliminate air artifacts.

Signal attenuation is another factor in the production of artifacts. Attenuation is a decrease in the amplitude and intensity of the ultrasound signal as the wave travels through a medium such as tissue. Attenuation may occur for any of three reasons: (1) conversion, in which sound is changed into heat; (2) reflection, in which some of the sound waves are returned from the boundary of a medium; and (3) scattering, which is the diffusion or redirection of sound in several directions (AIUM, 2014a, 2014b).

Refraction, reverberation, and mirror imaging are some other types of ultrasound artifacts. For example, a reverberation artifact occurs when a strong echo is returned to the transducer from a large acoustic interface (**FIGURE 2-9**). This echo bounces back to the same tissues, causing additional echoes parallel and equidistant to the first. Shadowing artifact occurs when the sound beam fails to pass through an object (e.g., a bone does not allow any sound to pass through it) and only a shadow is seen behind it (**FIGURE 2-10**).

Ultrasound operators can often minimize artifacts simply by manipulating the transducer. Artifacts, however, can be beneficial and essential for accurate diagnosis in some situations. For example, bone typically creates a shadow. In a fetus

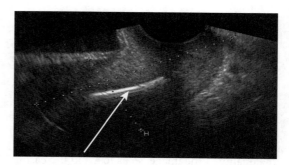

FIGURE 2-9 Reverberation of sound waves off of dense intrauterine device (IUD; appearing hyperechoic as a "double line") making structure look "thickened."

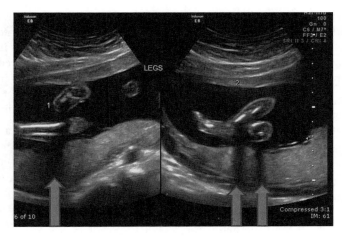

FIGURE 2-10 Acoustic shadowing, seen at the arrows.

with osteogenesis imperfecta, a strong shadow will not be present.

Artifacts may also be a product of the machine itself. There may be a problem with the internal electronics of the machine, such as a broken crystal in the head of the transducer or air bubbles trapped beneath the surface of the transducer membrane. These issues must be repaired by the manufacturer or someone qualified in ultrasound machine or transducer repair. Preventive maintenance and care of transducers adds to the longevity of the equipment and helps to maintain the quality of the image.

▶ Summary

Twenty-first century ultrasound technology has allowed us to obtain crystal clear images with relatively little effort, making the performance of ultrasound seemingly simple to incorporate into clinical practice, and with what may be misconstrued as minimal education and training requirements. However, as this chapter has described, potential bioeffects and harm may occur, thus mandating that all ultrasound users be familiar with ultrasound physics and the appropriate use of the technology. Ultrasound is a medical wonder; it should be reserved to improve quality and safety in patient care and not as yet another high-tech home entertainment device.

Study Questions

1. What do sound waves represent?
   a. Auditory vibrations
   b. Acoustic oscillations
   c. Acoustic static

2. Sound wave frequency is greater than:
   a. 20 Hz.
   b. 200 Hz.
   c. 20,000 Hz.

3. If the returning ultrasound signal has minimal echoes, what is it called?
   a. Isoechechoic
   b. Hyperechoic
   c. Hypoechoic

4. How is propagation of ultrasound energy is defined?
   a. Moving energy from deeper to more superficial anatomic structures
   b. Transmitting energy from one place to another
   c. Cooling the transmitted sound waves to reduced thermal power

5. Which type of tissue has the fastest propagation speed?
   a. Soft tissue
   b. Amniotic fluid
   c. Bone

6. Ultrasound transducers are differentiated from one another by their:
   a. weight.
   b. frequency.
   c. dynamic range.

7. How is frequency defined?
   a. Number of vibrations per unit of time
   b. Number of hertz per second
   c. Number of returning echoes per millisecond

8. How does frequency impact how sound waves are transmitted?
   a. The higher the frequency, the shorter the sound waves, and the better the resolution.
   b. The lower the frequency, the shorter the sound waves, and the better the resolution.
   c. The frequency does not impact how the sound waves are transmitted.

9. What is a benefit of a higher-frequency transducer?
   a. The sound waves will travel faster to deeper structures.
   b. Superficial anatomic structures will be visualized well.
   c. It generates less heat, thereby preventing it from having a thermal effect.

10. What is the piezoelectric element's function within the transducer?
    a. Converts electrical energy into mechanical energy
    b. Transmits and receives ultrasound waves
    c. Controls the frequency of the transducer

11. The transducer's resonant frequency depends on which aspect of the piezoelectric element?
    a. The shape
    b. The weight
    c. The thickness

12. A-mode ultrasound is which type of display mode?
    a. Multidimensional
    b. Single-dimensional
    c. Two-dimensional

13. B-mode display is which type of display mode?
    a. Brightness modulated, providing a cross-section of objects in real time
    b. Baseline modulated, providing a cross-section of objects in real time
    c. Brightness modulated, providing a cross-section in a single-dimensional static image

14. What is M-mode ultrasound?
    a. A graphic B-mode in multiple dimensions representing movement
    b. A graphic A-mode in a single dimension representing movement
    c. A graphic B-mode in a single dimension representing movement

15. What is the term for the returning echoes when the image appears dark with minimal but some reflected sound waves?
    a. Hypoechoic
    b. Anechoic
    c. Isoechoic

16. Which type of ultrasound allows for detection of blood flow through vessels?
    a. Continuous- and/or pulsed-wave Doppler
    b. Doppler shift
    c. Duplex Doppler

17. What should the choice of transducer be based upon?
    a. The density of the structure to be investigated
    b. The type of the structure to be investigated
    c. The depth of the structure to be investigated

18. What is the ideal range for transabdominal transducers in OB/GYN?
    a. 3–6 MHz
    b. 5–10 MHz
    c. 9–12 MHz

19. What do the terms "longitudinal" and "transverse" refer to in transabdominal imaging?
    a. The view of the structure obtained by the probe
    b. The view shown on the display monitor
    c. The relationship of the transducer to the anatomic structure

20. What do the terms "sagittal" and "coronal" refer to in transabdominal imaging?
    a. The view of the structure obtained by the probe
    b. The view shown on the display monitor
    c. The relationship of the transducer to the anatomic structure

21. Which scan planes are used with the transvaginal transducer orientation?
    a. Longitudinal and transverse
    b. Longitudinal and coronal
    c. Transverse and coronal

22. Which term is used to describe the bioeffect of tissue absorption of ultrasound waves?
    a. Mechanical
    b. Thermal
    c. Cavitation

23. What can be done to minimize the creation of cavitation?
    a. Limit output power
    b. Scan longer with lower power
    c. Use color Doppler

References

American Institute of Ultrasound in Medicine (AIUM). (2008). *Recommended ultrasound terminology* (3rd ed.). Laurel, MD: Author.

American Institute of Ultrasound in Medicine (AIUM). (2014a). AIUM as low as reasonably achievable (ALARA) principle. Retrieved from https://www.aium.org/officialStatements/39

American Institute of Ultrasound in Medicine (AIUM). (2014b). *Medical ultrasound safety* (3rd ed.). Laurel, MD: Author.

American Institute of Ultrasound in Medicine (AIUM). (2016a). Statement on measurement of fetal heart rate. Retrieved from https://www.aium.org/officialStatements/43

American Institute of Ultrasound in Medicine (AIUM). (2016b). Statement on the safe use of Doppler ultrasound during 11–14 week scans (or earlier in pregnancy). Retrieved from https://www.aium.org/officialStatements/42

American Institute of Ultrasound in Medicine (AIUM). (2018). Guidelines for cleaning and preparing external- and internal-use ultrasound probes between patients, safe handling, and use of ultrasound coupling gel. Retrieved from https://www.aium.org/officialStatements/57

Bahner, D. P., Blickendorf, M., Bockbrader, M., Adkins, E., Vira, A., Boulger, C., & Panchal, A. (2016). Language of transducer manipulation. *Journal of Ultrasound in Medicine, 35(1),* 183–188.

CHAPTER 3

Ultrasound in Gynecology and Reproductive Technologies

Three of the most common indications for point-of-care (POC) sonography in gynecology are perhaps the evaluation of the endometrial thickness, the measurement of follicles during ovarian stimulation with assisted reproductive technologies, and intrauterine device (IUD) insertions and/or localization. (**BOX 3-1**). In addition, sonography may be utilized to measure retained residual urine following birth and in uro-gynecologic bladder assessments. Sonograms are also performed following a successful assisted reproductive procedure for pregnancy confirmation (ASRM, 2009), which is included as part of a limited pelvic ultrasound examination, although sonography in the first trimester of pregnancy is discussed in the *Sonography in the First Trimester* chapter. This is by no means a complete list, as the indications for gynecologic ultrasound continue to grow as the technology's assessment and diagnostic utility in POC settings is further supported.

A more novel use of pelvic ultrasound in the educational setting is the use of sonography in teaching the bimanual examination in medical schools due to limited opportunities for medical students to practice these examinations (Parikh et al., 2018). It can assist in developing confidence in structure identification and physical examination skills. This educational concept applies equally to any advanced practice education and clinical training program and may be worthy of consideration. A screening pelvic ultrasound should be done prior to the use of human models, as noted in the *Guidelines, Education, and Professional Responsibility* chapter.

It is recommended that a standard pelvic sonogram be performed prior to any POC ultrasound whenever feasible. Following a complete pelvic sonogram, a "limited" or POC gynecologic ultrasound examination can be restricted to a specific organ or measurement (AIUM, 2017). OB/GYN advanced practice clinicians (APs) have already studied normal pelvic anatomy and physiology, and the logical next step is to transfer that knowledge to the sonographic appearance of female pelvic anatomy. The purpose of this chapter, therefore, is to describe the female reproductive anatomic structures as visualized by ultrasound, illustrate the sonographic measuring of these structures, and review the documentation and communication of both negative and positive findings.

▶ Ultrasound Anatomy of the Female Pelvis

The female pelvis can be imaged using the transabdominal (TA) or transvaginal (TV) approach. Transabdominal sonography (TAS) requires a full urinary bladder to displace the air-filled bowel from the lower abdomen and to provide an acoustic window through which to visualize the pelvic organs (**FIGURE 3-1**). An acoustic window is a structure that has no acoustic impedance (no returning ultrasound signals); it is referred to as anechoic. The absence of returning sound waves imparts a black image on the monitor. In addition, this lack of impedance allows for passage of sound and enhanced visualization of deeper structures. In the transabdominal approach, the depth of penetration into the body is much deeper when compared to the TV approach, so more structures can be accessed. However, the transabdominal transducer has inherently less resolution than the transvaginal approach.

Transvaginal sonography (TVS) requires an empty urinary bladder and is performed with high-frequency transducers. Use of higher frequency offers better resolution and, therefore, better visualization of the structures. However, the depth

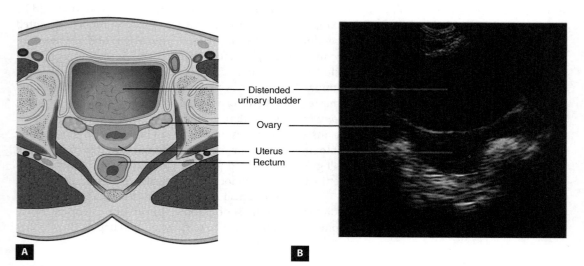

Distended urinary bladder

Ovary

Uterus
Rectum

A   **B**

FIGURE 3-1 Comparison of schematic anatomic structures with ultrasound image of transverse section of the female pelvis. **(A)** An anatomic section through the urinary bladder, uterus, and rectum. **(B)** Transverse ultrasound scan of same structures.

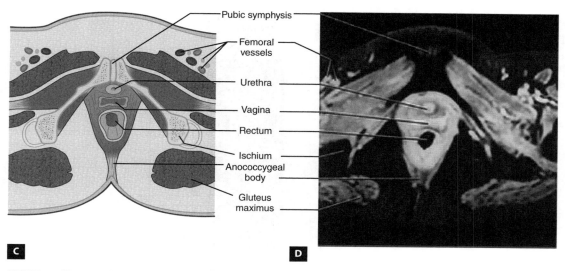

C

D

FIGURE 3-1 *(Continued)* **(C)** An anatomic section through the urethra, vagina, and rectum. **(D)** Transverse magnetic resonance image (MRI).

of penetration of a high-resolution transducer is shallower than that of a low-resolution transducer. For transvaginal ultrasound, this penetration depth is accomplished by literally getting physically closer to the structures by way of the tip of the vaginal wand being in close proximity to the structure being imaged. In many circumstances, it is helpful to use both TA and TVS to visualize the entire pelvis.

Urinary Bladder

The urinary bladder is an important landmark in identifying pelvic anatomy. The bladder walls are composed of a thick (detrusor) muscle that is lined with a thin mucosa and covered externally by a serosal layer. This thickness or density reflects sound waves, which appear "whiter" than the black anechoic appearance of the fluid-filled bladder, thereby creating an easily distinguishable outline of the bladder.

Bladder distention causes a thinning and stretching of the bladder wall, which then appears as a thin echogenic line. With partial distention, the detrusor muscle is relaxed and appears as a hypoechoic layer around the inner mucosa (**FIGURE 3-2**). The ureters can be recognized when they are abnormally filled with fluid. They can be distinguished from the adjacent iliac vessels by their more echogenic walls,

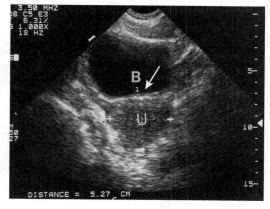

FIGURE 3-2 Distended bladder (B) showing the detrusor muscle at the arrow, and the uterus (U).

by their anatomic path, and by color Doppler. A urine jet can be seen in grayscale or color Doppler as the ureters enter into the posterior portion of the bladder.

Pelvic Musculature

On ultrasound, muscles appear as hypoechoic bands of tissue, with low-level echoes and thin, linear hyperechoic striations. The skeletal muscles of the false pelvis include the rectus and transverse abdominis and the iliopsoas muscles (**FIGURES 3-3** and **3-4**).

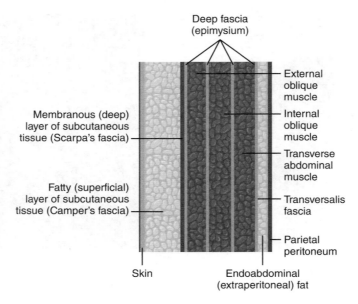

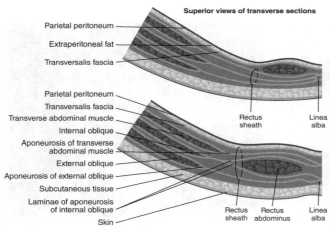

FIGURE 3-3 Longitudinal and transverse sections of the abdominal wall, showing the rectus abdominis muscle and the contributions of the lateral abdominal muscles to its sheath.

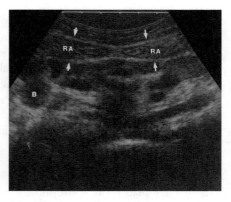

FIGURE 3-4 Transverse image of the anterior abdominal wall, showing the rectus abdominus muscle (RA), the anterior and posterior rectus sheath (arrows), and loops of bowel (B) in the abdominal cavity.

The muscles of the true pelvis include the obturator internus muscles, the piriformis muscles, and the muscles of the pelvic diaphragm. The last are composed of three paired muscles—the coccygeus, the pubococcygeus, and the iliococcygeus—which form the floor of the true pelvis and support the pelvic organs (**FIGURES 3-5** and **3-6**).

The pubococcygeus and iliococcygeus muscles together form the levator ani muscles (**FIGURE 3-7**). The iliopsoas muscles can be identified in the sagittal

(longitudinal) view as linear structures along the pelvic sidewall that are medial and slightly anterior to the iliacus muscles and as ovoid structures that are anterior and lateral to the urinary bladder on transverse imaging (**FIGURE 3-8**).

The obturator internus muscles run parallel to the lateral walls of the bladder on transverse scans, but they are more difficult to identify in the sagittal plane. The muscles of the pelvic diaphragm are seen best in the transverse plane at the level of the cervix.

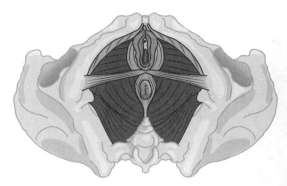

FIGURE 3-5 Pelvic floor muscles as seen from below in the supine female subject. The muscles of the pelvic diaphragm are dark gray and the associated pelvic muscles are light gray.

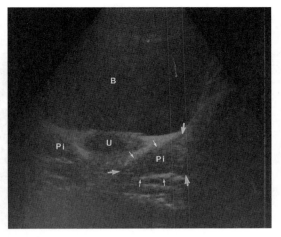

FIGURE 3-6 Transverse transabdominal image through a full bladder (B) showing the uterus (U) and the piriformis muscles (Pi) within the arrows, posterior to the cervix.

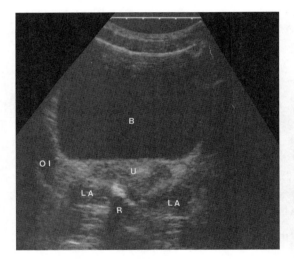

FIGURE 3-7 Transverse transabdominal image of the levator ani (LA) muscles, the right obturator internus muscle (OI), the bladder (B), and the rectum (R), posterior to the cervix.

Many pelvic muscles are difficult to evaluate sonographically. It is not unusual for normal muscles to be mistaken for free fluid, a mass, or other pathology; therefore, it is important to recognize the appearance of muscles, to know where they attach, and to understand how the muscle is oriented.

Pelvic Vasculature

The common iliac arteries branch into the internal and external arteries. The internal and external iliac veins join to form the common iliac vein. The

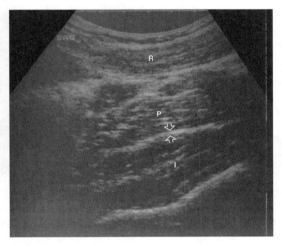

FIGURE 3-8 Sagittal transabdominal image with the transducer angled laterally to demonstrate the long axis of the psoas major (P), and the iliacus muscles (I), with interposed fascial plan (open arrows).

internal iliac vessels lie posterior and slightly lateral to the ovaries and are important landmarks to help identify and locate the ovaries (**FIGURE 3-9**), especially when the ovaries are small and lack follicles.

The internal iliac arteries have a width of 5 to 7 mm and are pulsatile, whereas the veins are typically larger (1 cm), more medially located, and do not pulsate. The blood supply to the uterus and

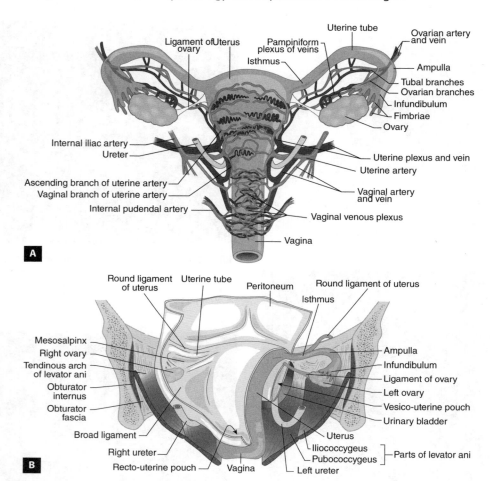

FIGURE 3-9 Broad ligament and blood supply of the uterus, vagina, and ovaries.

vagina is provided via the uterine artery, which is a branch of the internal iliac artery (**FIGURE 3-10**).

The uterine arteries give rise to the arcuate arteries, which encircle the uterus and branch into the radial arteries. The radial arteries pass through the myometrium, become the straight arteries at the level of the endometrium, and then branch to form the spiral arteries. The blood supply to the endometrium is provided by the straight and spiral arteries, with the latter being responsive to hormonal changes of the menstrual cycle. The ovarian blood supply comes from both the ovarian and uterine artery and vein. The ovarian artery enters the ovarian hilum via the mesovarium, while the uterine artery reaches the ovarian hilum via the broad ligament.

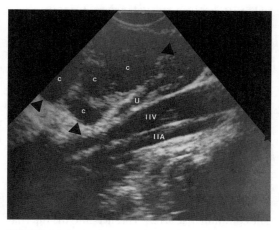

FIGURE 3-10 Sagittal transvaginal scan of left internal iliac artery (IIA) and vein (IIV) posterior to the ovary (arrows).

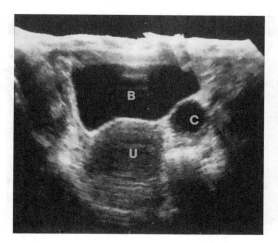

FIGURE 3-11 Transverse transabdominal image showing the anechoic distended bladder (B), uterus (U), and smooth-walled anechoic corpus luteum cyst (C) in the left ovary.

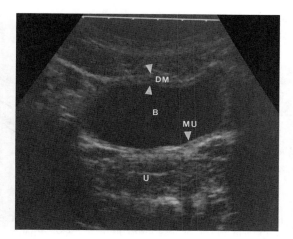

FIGURE 3-12 Transverse transabdominal scan of a partially distended bladder (B) and uterus (U) showing the relaxed detrusor muscle (DM) surrounding the inner mucosal layer (MU).

Uterus

The uterus is the most prominent landmark in the pelvis. It can be visualized by both transabdominal and transvaginal ultrasound (**FIGURES 3-11** and **3-12**). In the nonpregnant uterus, the cervix represents approximately one-third to one-half of the total uterine length, and it is approximately twice the diameter of the corpus. The adult uterus is approximately 6 to 8 cm in length and 3 to 5 cm wide.

The typical uterine position is anteverted, although a full bladder will displace an anteverted uterus into a more horizontal position (**FIGURE 3-13**). Variations include the following (**FIGURES 3-14** and **3-15**):

- Retroverted uterus, which is the posterior angulation of the uterus and cervix relative to the vagina
- Retroflexed uterus, which describes the posterior angulation of the uterine corpus relative to the cervix
- Anteflexed uterus, which is the anterior angulation of the uterine corpus relative to the cervix.

Myometrium

The myometrium, which exhibits medium- to low-level homogeneous echoes, can be distinguished

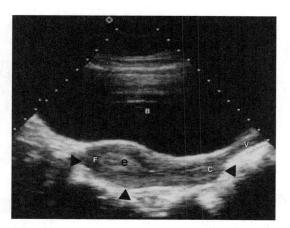

FIGURE 3-13 Transabdominal midline sagittal image of the anteverted uterus (within black arrowheads), viewed through a distended anechoic urinary bladder (B). The endometrium (e) can be distinguished from the surrounding myometrium. F = fundus, C = cervix, V = vagina.

from the endometrium, which varies in thickness and echogenicity throughout the menstrual cycle. Uterine blood vessels can be imaged using both transabdominal and transvaginal sonography. When seen, the arcuate arteries appear as anechoic tubular structures at the periphery of the myometrium. Calcifications may be seen within the arcuate arteries of elderly patients and appear as echogenic foci along the periphery of the uterus.

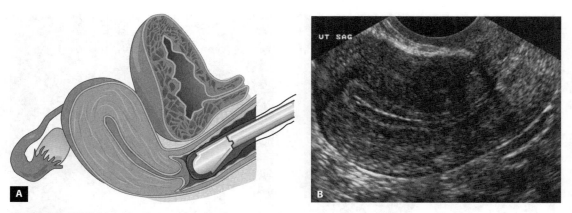

FIGURE 3-14 **(A)** Schematic of vaginal probe directed in the sagittal view of anteflexed uterus. **(B)** Transvaginal sagittal image of the anteflexed uterus in the schematic.

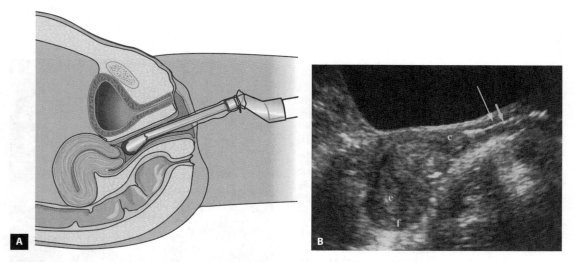

FIGURE 3-15 **(A)** Vaginal-directed schematic of sagittal view of retroflexed uterus. **(B)** Transvaginal sagittal image comparison with the schematic of the retroflexed uterus. White arrows point to the vagina, which appears elongated secondary to a full bladder. Repeating the scan with an empty bladder would be recommended.

Endometrium

The endometrium is composed of basal and functional layers. Changes occur in the uterus in response to estradiol fluctuations, which are reflected in the overall uterine volume and in the thickness and echogenicity of the endometrium.

After menses, the endometrium appears as a thin echogenic stripe. During the follicular phase, the endometrial thickness gradually increases as the endometrium proliferates. The endometrium then appears as a triple-line or trilaminar complex composed of the interfaces between the myometrium, the endometrium, and the central midline stripe. After ovulation, the secretory endometrium appears thicker and more echogenic (**FIGURE 3-16**).

When a woman presents during the perimenopausal or postmenopausal time frame with a chief complaint of abnormal uterine bleeding, evaluation will most likely include a pelvic ultrasound, often specifically to measure the endometrium (American College of Nurse-Midwives [ACNM], 2016).

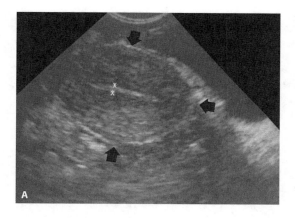

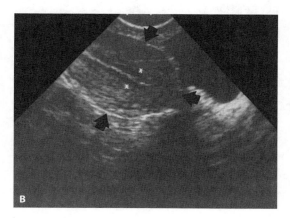

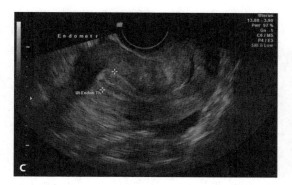

FIGURE 3-16 Changes in the endometrium during the menstrual cycle. **(A)** Early follicular phase after menses showing the uterus (arrows) and the endometrium (white "line" between stars). **(B)** Late proliferative phase, showing the typical triple-line of the endometrium (white line between "stars") and the uterus (arrows). **(C)** Early secretory phase, showing the endometrium (between the white + signs).

To measure the endometrial thickness, the endometrium should be sonographically viewed in the sagittal plane with a continuous view from the cervix to the fundus. The measurement should include both layers of the endometrium (ACOG, 2018; Tsuda, 2018). Place the calipers at the bright leading edge, and measure to the bright far edge as noted in Figure 3-16.

The incidence of malignancy in women with postmenopausal bleeding ranges from 1% to 14%. Transvaginal sonography should be the first diagnostic test in such a case because of the extremely high negative predictive value of a thin echogenic endometrial stripe. Women with postmenopausal bleeding with an endometrial measurement of 4 mm or less have a risk of malignancy of 1/917; such a finding reliably excludes endometrial carcinoma. If the endometrial thickness is greater than 4 to 5 mm in a symptomatic postmenopausal woman, pathology cannot be ruled out (ACOG, 2018; Goldstein, 2012). In some women, visualization may not be adequate and sonohysterography with transvaginal sonography may be needed to visualize the endometrial cavity (**FIGURE 3-17**).

Cervix and Vagina

The cervix can be visualized with transvaginal sonography. During transvaginal scanning, the transducer should be placed at or near the external os.

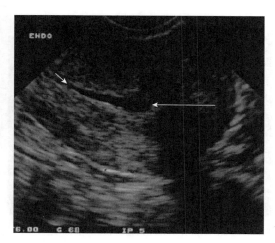

FIGURE 3-17 Sonohysterography showing normal uterine cavity (anechoic area between white arrows).

This allows for optimal visualization of the cervix as well as the uterus. If the vagina needs to be imaged, the transducer can be partially withdrawn. Mucus within the cervical canal appears echogenic, except during the periovulatory period, when it contains more fluid and appears hypoechoic (**FIGURE 3-18**). Small inclusion (nabothian) cysts are frequently seen within the muscle of the cervix at the region of the cervical canal. They appear as thin-walled hypoechoic structures, usually less than 1 cm in size. Measurement of cervical length is discussed in the *Point-of-Care Sonography in the Second Trimester* chapter.

On transabdominal examination, the vagina can be seen immediately posterior to the bladder neck.

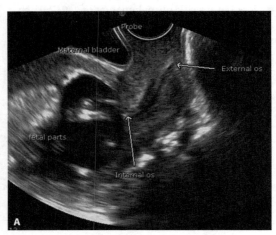

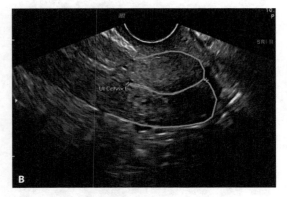

FIGURE 3-18 **(A)** Internal and external cervical os. **(B)** Cervical length with the cervix outlined.

From B. K. Taylor.

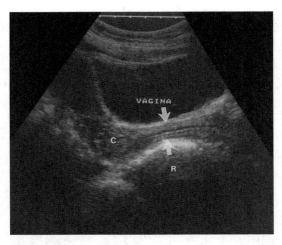

FIGURE 3-19 Midline sagittal transabdominal image of the vagina (between white arrows) with the black stripe indicating the cervical canal. The vagina is anterior to the rectum (R), posterior to the bladder, and inferior to the cervix (C).

It appears as a collapsed tube exhibiting low-level echoes, with a strong central echo from the apposed surfaces of the vaginal mucosa (**FIGURE 3-19**).

Pelvic Adnexa

Bowel

The sonographic appearance of the bowel depends on the amount of fluid, gas, and fecal material within its lumen (**FIGURE 3-20**). Loops of small bowel can be seen around the uterus and ovaries during transvaginal scanning, often showing peristalsis.

Gas in the small intestine can sometimes obscure adequate visualization of the ovaries. The sigmoid colon and rectum frequently appear echogenic, with posterior-wall shadowing from gas and fecal contents. The peristaltic activity demonstrated in the small bowel is not seen in the sigmoid colon and rectum; nevertheless, this peristalsis can sometimes help to discriminate a pelvic mass from other structures.

Fallopian Tubes

Normal fallopian tubes, which measure approximately 10 cm in length, are not routinely identified through ultrasonography. Because they are small

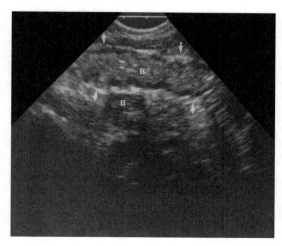

FIGURE 3-20 Transvaginal coronal image of a loop of the small intestine (B = bowel) surrounded by arrows, demonstrating submucosal folds and echogenic bowel contents.

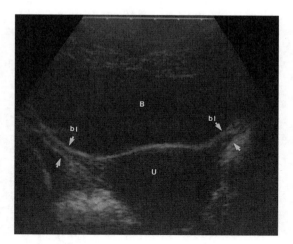

FIGURE 3-21 Transverse transabdominal image of the uterus at the level of the fundus (white arrow at the echogenic "line"). The broad ligament (bl) is seen as a tubular structure extending laterally from the uterine cornua (between the arrows). Normal fallopian tubes are not routinely identified on ultrasonography. The bladder (B) and uterus (U) are also identified.

and tortuous, they can be difficult to distinguish from the broad ligament, which appears as a band of low-level echoes extending from the uterine cornua lateral to the ovaries (**FIGURE 3-21**).

Ovaries

The ovaries are usually located between the uterine fundus and the pelvic sidewall, medial to the iliopsoas muscles and external iliac vessels, and anterior to the internal iliac vessels. However, the precise location of the ovaries may vary, and they may be identified in the cul-de-sac or above the uterine fundus. Sonographically, the ovaries appear as distinct ovoid structures, slightly less echogenic or isoechoic than the myometrium, and contain follicles in premenopausal women (**FIGURE 3-22**). The internal iliac vessels also serve as useful ovarian landmarks, especially after menopause, when ovaries are small and devoid of follicles (**FIGURE 3-23**).

When the transabdominal approach is used, a full bladder is necessary to visualize the ovaries in the sagittal and transverse planes. Gentle pressure can be applied to the abdominal wall to displace the bowel and optimize visualization of each ovary. When the bladder is full, it can be used as an acoustic window to better evaluate the ovary. For example, when imaging the right ovary, slide the transducer toward the patient's left side and angle it through the bladder to the right ovary. Transvaginal imaging of the ovary may be difficult if bowel shadowing is excessive, if the ovaries are displaced, or if the ovaries are small (as is the case in postmenopausal women). Imaging the ovaries may be challenging.

The entire adnexa should be evaluated for free fluid, masses, or cysts. To identify the ovaries using TVS, begin in a coronal plane near the cornu of the uterus. Follow the broad ligament into the adnexa to the ovary. Scan the ovary in the coronal plane by angling the transducer from anterior to posterior. In the sagittal plane, images are obtained by angling the transducer from lateral (at the iliac vessels) to medial (back to the uterus). The ovaries are usually located posterior and lateral to the uterus, anterior to the internal iliac artery and vein, and medial to the external iliac vessels. The iliac vessels provide an anatomic landmark for localization of the ovaries, and color flow Doppler can be useful in locating the vessels as landmarks.

Ovarian size is expressed in terms of ovarian volume, which is calculated using the formula for

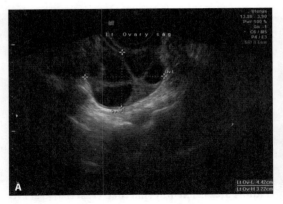 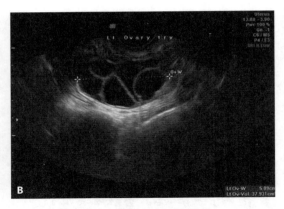

FIGURE 3-22 Ovarian measurements. **(A)** Transvaginal sagittal scan of left ovary length and width. **(B)** Transverse view of same ovary showing view for determining width. Multiple follicles such as these are usually the result of ovarian stimulation for assisted reproduction.

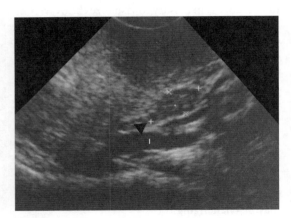

FIGURE 3-23 Transvaginal sagittal image of a postmenopausal ovary (between + signs). The iliac (i) vessels help to identify the ovary when it is small with few visible follicles (black arrowhead).

a prolate ellipse (length × width × height × 0.523) (**FIGURE 3-24**). Ovarian size increases throughout childhood and puberty, and it fluctuates across the menstrual cycle in association with growth and ovulation of the dominant follicle. Ovarian volume decreases after menopause.

Ovarian volume and follicular number are essential ultrasound diagnostic criteria for polycystic ovary syndrome (PCOS) (**FIGURE 3-25**). PCOS affects 6% to 10% of all women and often starts in adolescence. The Rotterdam Criteria define

ovaries as polycystic if there are 12 or more follicles measuring 2 to 9 mm (FNPS = follicle number per single cross-section of the ovary) and/or ovarian volume (OV) greater than 10 cm³ (Rosen, 2008). Since 2003, however, questions about these criteria have arisen, as many normal women meet them. A study done by Lujan et al. (2013) with Cornell University and Canadian researchers demonstrated a higher diagnostic sensitivity when total number of follicles per *ovary* (FNPO), using multisector or three-dimensional scanning, exceeds 2. Although ovarian volume has been considered a hallmark diagnostic criterion, Atiomo et al. (2000) found the following findings were more sensitive as diagnostic criteria for PCOS than ovarian volume: (1) 10 or more follicles per ovary, (2) peripheral distribution of follicles, and (3) stromal brightness. PCOS is the most common cause of irregular menses and the most common cause of infertility in women, and ultrasonography is a critical tool in providing for its early detection and management (Lujan et al., 2013; Williams, Mortada, & Porter, 2016).

Ovarian Response to Assisted Reproductive Procedures. When assisted reproductive technologies and ovary-stimulating medications are being utilized, production of multiple follicles can occur. This follicular growth is followed clinically by serial sonographic measurements. Because

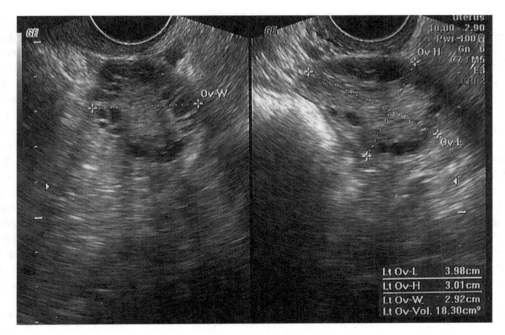

FIGURE 3-24 These images demonstrate the measurements needed to obtain the ovarian volume (between + signs). Note that more than 10 follicles are present on each ovary.

Image courtesy of Diana Dowdy personal collection.

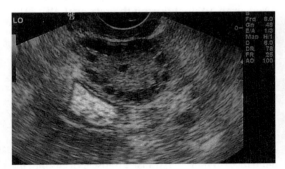

FIGURE 3-25 Multiple follicles noted around the periphery of the ovary with polycystic ovary syndrome. Follicles appear numerous and are easily imaged.

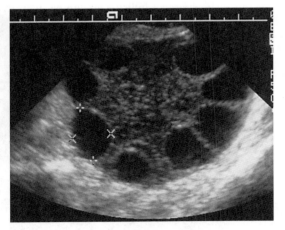

FIGURE 3-26 Multiple ovarian follicles (approximately nine) that have been induced by ovary-stimulating medication in assisted reproductive medicine, with measurement of one follicle at the cursors.

follicles are filled with fluid, they appear anechoic (**FIGURE 3-26**).

There is a close correlation between increasing levels of estradiol and the increasing size of the dominant follicle, as estimated by measurements of mean follicle diameter or total surface area. There is also a close correlation between estimated follicular volume by ultrasound and that assessed at the time of laparoscopy. Although follicular growth and ovulation can be determined with great accuracy, the use of follicle size alone as an absolute predictor of ovulation is limited because of variation in follicle size at rupture. Other sonographic findings may help to predict imminent ovulation more precisely. These include the "double contour" sign, which represents separation of the theca layer from the granulosa cell layer, and visualization of the cumulus oophorus 12 to 24 hours prior to ovulation (**FIGURE 3-27**).

With assisted reproductive technologies, the follicular number and interval growth are followed closely with both hormone levels and sonographic imaging. Once the ovary is identified, the ovarian size (length, anterior–posterior [AP], and transverse) is determined. All follicles, cysts, or masses should be noted. Follicles are measured in two dimensions at the largest diameter (Rosen et al., 2008).

With in vitro fertilization, the goal is to induce multiple follicles in each ovary. During the normal or non-induced cycle, generally only a single follicle dominates and enlarges while the oocyte inside matures. A follicular measurement of greater than 18 mm is considered to contain a mature egg. According to Rosen et al. (2008), the odds of a mature oocyte resulting from a 16- to 18-mm follicle size are 37% when compared to a follicle measuring more than 18 mm. More recently, Abbara (2018) enlarged the range showing that follicles containing mature oocytes measured from between 12 mm to 19 mm.

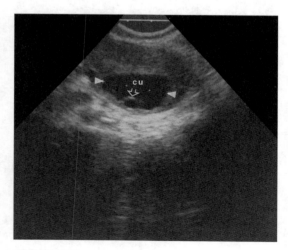

FIGURE 3-27 Transvaginal section of an ovary with a preovulatory follicle (arrowheads) of 28 mm. The cumulus oophorous (cu) can be seen projecting from the wall of the follicle into the follicular fluid (arrow).

The odds of oocyte maturity decrease progressively with decreasing follicular size. Any follicle greater than 10 mm should be measured and documented. If multiple follicles are present, as in a stimulated in vitro fertilization cycle, the largest follicles should be measured, and the total number of follicles documented according to established protocol (AIUM, 2017).

After follicular collapse, the corpus luteum appears as a hypoechoic structure with irregular walls and internal echoes. Thereafter, the size and general appearance of the corpus luteum are variable. The structure may enlarge and fill with echogenic material corresponding to fresh hemorrhagic material. Over time, it can organize to produce a complex pattern of cystic areas and solid strands (**FIGURE 3-28**). There is no relationship between the size and appearance of the corpus luteum and progesterone secretion. With color Doppler, a ring of color may be noted around a corpus luteum.

Sonography is also crucial in the retrieval of the oocytes in assisted reproduction. The reproductive medicine physician uses a transvaginal ultrasound probe fitted with a retrieval needle. Transabdominal ultrasound guidance may be used as an adjunct during the retrieval. With the patient lightly sedated, the transvaginal ultrasound transducer is used to identify each follicle. The retrieval needle is then advanced into each follicle, and the fluid and oocyte are aspirated with gentle suction. The contents are collected in a small tube, and the process of oocyte identification and assessment begins.

With successful fertilization of the ovum or ova, sonography may also be used to assist with the guidance of embryo(s) transfer transcervically into the endometrial cavity. The catheter used for insertion of the embryo(s) is easily seen with the transabdominal transducer (AIUM, 2017; ASRM, 2017).

Use of Color Doppler. Color Doppler and pulsed-wave Doppler can be used to evaluate changes in pelvic blood flow across the ovulatory cycle. The Doppler classification is based on the presence and duration or absence of diastolic flow in the pelvic arteries.

Doppler ultrasound has also assumed a significant role in the evaluation of the ovaries in

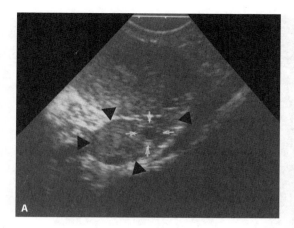

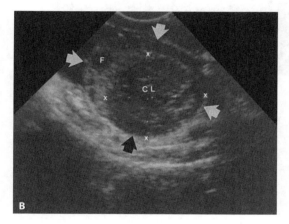

FIGURE 3-28 **(A)** A sagittal section of the ovary (black arrow heads) after follicle rupture, showing the variable appearance of a corpus luteum (white arrows). **(B)** Circumferential measurement (at Xs) of a cystic corpus luteum (CL) containing echogenic hemorrhagic material and another follicile (F). Arrows indicate ovarian tissue.

(ASRM, 2008, Zatel 2000). This can be beneficial when differentiating a tubo-ovarian abscess from a hydrosalpinx.

▶ Sonographic Localization of Intrauterine Devices

Many providers use ultrasound to assist with the insertion of IUDs (Nowitzki, 2015). Transvaginal assessment of uterine size and position may be done prior to insertion, as well as to verify or confirm IUD placement after the device's insertion (**FIGURES 3-29** and **3-30**). If on subsequent examinations the IUD string is not palpable or cannot be seen on speculum exam, the IUD location may be determined sonographically.

For a number of reasons, ultrasound is the recommended initial imaging modality in IUD localization: Sonography equipment is generally readily available; this technology has a lower cost than other imaging modalities; it avoids ionizing radiation and radiation concerns; and ultrasound is minimally invasive in nature. If the IUD cannot be seen with point-of-care TVS, a standard (complete) pelvic ultrasound examination is warranted, often to include three-dimensional (3-D) volume assessments. Three-dimensional imaging can

perimenopausal women as well as menopausal women. Superimposed color Doppler imaging of the ovaries allows possible detection of normal, suspicious, and pathologic blood flow characteristics in the blood vessels, which helps distinguish between benign and malignant lesions (ASRM, 2008). Additionally, Doppler can assist in characterization of adnexal masses, such as tubo-ovarian abscess

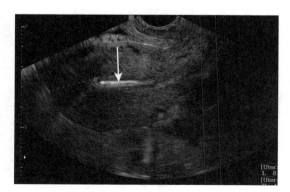

FIGURE 3-29 Sagittal image of the uterine cavity with an IUD (hyperechoic area) at arrow.

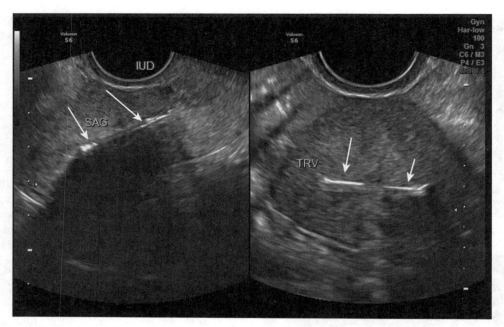

FIGURE 3-30 The IUD is noted to be in the endometrial canal within the uterus. The IUD (the hyperechoic bright white "line" at the arrow) is seen in the sagittal as well as transverse planes.)

sometimes aid in identifying IUD malposition within the endometrium or myometrium. If the IUD has migrated outside the uterine cavity into the bowel, bowel cavity, or bladder, sonographic visualization of the IUD can be difficult due to bowel gas (Nilsestuen, 2013). If the IUD cannot be identified sonographically, a plain film of the abdomen may be beneficial.

▶ Sonographic Assessment of the Bladder

There are several clinical indications for the sonographic assessment of bladder urine volume in both men and women (Abdelwahab, Abdalla, Sherief, Ibrahim, & Shamaa, 2014). Perhaps the most common indication in women is during the uro-gynecologic workup for complaints such as bladder leakage or retention issues. It can also be very informative during the postpartum period

when there is concern about inability to void or to completely empty the bladder (AIUM, 2014).

▶ Documentation and Subsequent Care

All findings from a POC sonogram should be documented in the medical record. Based on pelvic ultrasound guidelines, all POC sonograms performed in conjunction with reproductive medicine technologies or women's healthcare assessment should include specific information about each anatomic structure. Some structures, such as ovarian follicles or endometrial thickness, require measurements. All of the findings need to be documented.

Since a POC sonogram is generally neither a diagnostic nor a comprehensive pelvic ultrasound examination, recommendations also exist for the appropriate timing for comprehensive pelvic ultrasound. In reproductive medicine, it is advised that a comprehensive pelvic ultrasound to assess for pelvic pathology be performed 4 to 6 months *prior* to the beginning of a stimulated cycle (AIUM, 2017). Any POC sonogram performed for a specific gynecologic complaint may also warrant follow-up with a comprehensive scan.

Gynecologic and POC pelvic sonograms performed by nurses, midwives, or advanced practice nurses should be done with appropriate direct or indirect physician supervision and the availability of consultation and collaboration (ACNM, 2018; AWHONN, 2016). The definition of "supervision" may vary depending on state laws and institutional policies. Nonetheless, a preestablished means of communicating findings or inconclusive results should be determined and clarified, and a line of contact established for physician consultation and collaboration (ACNM, 2018; AWHONN, 2016).

▶ Summary

Nurses and advanced practitioners in women's health care who have received the appropriate education and training may perform some or all of the components of the pelvic ultrasound examination based on institutional policies and procedures, the scope of practice, and laws within the state. Each type of pelvic sonogram does have established guidelines that should be followed for each specific procedure, as well as a format for comprehensive documentation and communication of findings.

Study Questions

1. Why is a fluid-filled bladder recommended when performing a gynecologic transabdominal ultrasound exam?
   a. To displace the air-filled bowel from the lower abdomen and to provide an acoustic window through which to visualize the pelvic organs
   b. To prevent mirror-image artifact from sound waves scattering off of denser tissue
   c. To displace the bowel, which may have fecal matter that can cause a reverberation of sound waves

2. What is the difference in frequency between a transvaginal (TV) and a transabdominal (TA) ultrasound transducer?
   a. They are the same frequency.
   b. The TA is a higher frequency than the TV.
   c. The TV is a higher frequency than the TA.

3. Why are the internal iliac vessels (IIVs) used to help identify the ovaries?
   a. The IIVs are easily visualized and lie posterior and slightly lateral to the ovaries.
   b. The ovaries are very difficult to visualize when they contain cysts or follicles.
   c. The IIVs are not easily visualized, so if they can be seen, the ovaries will be adjacent to them.

4. Why should the bladder be empty when doing a transvaginal pelvic scan?
   a. It is too uncomfortable for the woman when the TV probe is placed.
   b. A full bladder will displace an anteverted uterus into a horizontal position.
   c. A full bladder will cause scattering of the sound waves.

5. How do the echoes returning from the myometrium appear?
   a. Medium- to low-level homogeneous echoes
   b. High echoes
   c. Consistently low echoes

6. How do the echoes returning from the endometrium of appear throughout the menstrual cycle?
   a. Consistently low echoes because the endometrium lacks density
   b. Consistently high echoes because the echoes traverse the myometrium
   c. The endometrium varies in thickness, so echogenicity varies throughout the menstrual cycle

7. When will the endometrium appear as a triple-line or trilaminar complex composed of the interfaces between the myometrium, the endometrium, and the central midline stripe?
   a. After menstruation has ended for that cycle
   b. During the follicular phase
   c. During menopause

8. In which plane is the endometrial thickness measured?
   a. In the sagittal plane, with a continuous view from the cervix to the fundus
   b. In the horizontal plane, with a full view of the width of the uterus
   c. With the transducer longitudinal to the endometrium, visualizing the entire endometrium

9. Why is transvaginal sonography of the endometrium the first diagnostic testing for endometrial cancer?
   a. It is noninvasive and has a high positive predictive value when a thick endometrium is noted.
   b. It has a high negative predictive value if a thin hyperechogenic stripe is present.
   c. It has a high negative predictive value if a thin echogenic endometrial stripe is present.

10. How does mucus within the cervical canal appear with the TV transducer?
    a. Echogenic, except during the periovulatory period, when it contains more fluid and appears hypoechoic.
    b. Consistently isoechoic throughout the cycle.
    c. Mucus cannot be visualized unless there is cervical dilation.

11. How will the vagina appear on a transabdominal examination?
    a. As an elongated tube, reflecting high-level echoes with a strong central echo from the uterus.
    b. As a collapsed tube, exhibiting low-level echoes with a strong central echo from the apposed surfaces of the vaginal mucosa.
    c. The vagina cannot be visualized with the transabdominal transducer because the full bladder obliterates it.

12. Which kind of artifact may result from the posterior wall of the colon if gas and fecal material are present?
    a. Mirroring
    b. Reverberation
    c. Shadowing

13. What is the sonographic appearance of normal fallopian tubes?
    a. They appear similar to a long tube with hyperechoic signals due to the dense tissue.
    b. They appear as fluid-filled hypoechoic elongated structures.
    c. They are not routinely identified.

14. How do the ovaries appear sonographically?
    a. As distinct ovoid structures, which are slightly less echogenic or isoechoic than the myometrium.
    b. They cannot be distinguished from the surrounding adnexa unless follicles, cysts, or other masses are present.
    c. As dense ovoid structures, which are much more echogenic than the endometrium.

15. Even though follicular growth and ovulation can be assessed with great accuracy during an assisted reproductive cycle, why is the use of follicle size alone as an absolute predictor of ovulation limited in predictive value?
    a. There is an unpredictable variation in follicle size at rupture.
    b. The number of follicles is a better predictor of pending ovulation.
    c. The larger follicles may not contain an ovum.

16. How are follicles measured for changes in growth in an assisted reproductive cycle?
    a. Follicles are measured in two dimensions at the largest diameter.
    b. Follicular circumference is measured using the ellipse.
    c. The anterior–posterior diameter is determined.

17. How does the corpus luteum appear after ovulation and/or collapse?
    a. Isoechoic and elliptical in shape, with hypoechoic signals returning from the fluid in the cul-de-sac.
    b. Initially only as a mixed echoic mass lateral to the ovary, and ultimately as only a fluid-filled cul-de-sac
    c. Initially as a hypoechoic structure with irregular walls and internal echoes with variable size and general appearance

18. Why is ultrasound the recommended initial imaging modality of choice in IUD localization?
    a. It uses non-ionizing radiation, which is drawn to the IUD, producing hyperechoic signals.
    b. It is minimally invasive in nature and is highly successful in visualizing the IUD.
    c. It is generally readily available and inexpensive, even though it does not have a high predictive value in determining the precise location of the IUD when seen.

19. What is the recommendation for pelvic assessment following a point-of-care (POC) sonogram performed by an AP or nurse?
    a. There is no further recommendation unless the results of the POC sonogram indicate the need for follow-up.
    b. A screening comprehensive pelvic ultrasound should be performed prior to the beginning of an assisted reproductive cycle or following any POC scan if one has never been done.
    c. A bimanual exam is needed to confirm the result of the POC scan.

20. Which means of communication is recommended when APs. assume the responsibility for performing POC ultrasound?
    a. A preestablished means for communicating findings or consulting regarding inconclusive results should be determined.
    b. It is up to the discretion of the PCA in all 50 states to determine when a consultation is necessary.
    c. It most states, only positive findings need to be conveyed to a collaborating or consulting physician.

21. In which clinical situations may transabdominal POC scan may be used to determine residual urine in the bladder?
    a. To determine if the source of "vaginal" discharge is vaginal or urine
    b. Whenever the chief complaint is suspicious for bladder infection
    c. To determine if urine remains in the bladder after voiding

References

Abbara, A., Vuong, L. N., Ho, V. N. A., Clarke, S. A., Jeffers, L., Comninos, A. N., . . . Dhillo, W. S. (2018). Measuring follicle size on day of trigger most likely to yield a mature oocyte. *Frontiers in Endocrinology, 9*, 193. doi: 10.3389/fendo.2018.00193

Abdelwahab, H. A., Abdalla, H. M., Sherief, M. H., Ibrahim, M. B., & Shamaa, M. A. (2014). The reliability and reproducibility of ultrasonography for measuring the residual urine volume in men with lower urinary tract symptoms. *Arab Journal of Urology, 12*(4), 285–289.

American College of Nurse-Midwives (ACNM). (2016). *Clinical Bulletin #15: Abnormal uterine bleeding.* Washington, DC: Author.

American College of Nurse-Midwives (ACNM). (2018). *Midwives performance of ultrasound in clinical practice.* Washington, DC: Author.

American College of Obstetricians and Gynecologists (ACOG). (2018). *The role of transvaginal ultrasonography in the evaluation of postmenopausal bleeding. Committee Opinion #734.* Washington, DC: Author.

American Institute of Ultrasound in Medicine (AIUM). (2014). *Practice guideline for the performance of ultrasound examinations of the female pelvis.* Laurel, MD: Author.

American Institute of Ultrasound in Medicine (AIUM). (2017). *Practice guideline: Ultrasound of the female pelvis for infertility and reproductive medicine.* Laurel, MD: Author

American Society for Reproductive Medicine (ASRM). (2008). Use of exogenous gonadotropins in anovulatory women (Practice Committee Technical Bulletin). *Fertility and Sterility, 90*, S7–S12.

American Society for Reproductive Medicine (ASRM). (2009). Position statement on nurses performing focused ultrasound examinations in a gynecology/infertility setting. Retrieved from https://www.asrm.org/globalassets/asrm/asrm-content/news-and-publications/practice-guidelines/for-non-members/position_statement_on_nurses_performing_focused_ultrasound-noprint.pdf

American Society for Reproductive Medicine (ASRM). (2017). Performing the embryo transfer: a guideline. Practice Committee of the American Society for Reproductive Medicine. *Fertility and Sterility, 107*, 882–896.

Association of Women's Health, Obstetric, and Neonatal Nurses (AWHONN). (2016). *Ultrasound examinations performed by registered nurses in obstetric, gynecologic, and reproductive medicine settings: Clinical competencies and education guide* (4th ed.). Washington, DC: Author.

Atiomo, W. U., Pearson, S., Shaw, S., Prentice, A., & Dubbins, P. (2000) Ultrasound criteria in the diagnosis of polycystic ovary syndrome (PCOS). *Ultrasound in Medicine and Biology, 26*(6), 977–980.

Goldstein, S. R. (2012). Sonography in postmenopausal bleeding. *Journal of Ultrasound in Medicine, 31*, 333–336.

Lujan, M. E., Jarrett, B. Y., Brooks, E. D., Reines, J. K., Peppin, A. K., Muhn, N., . . . Chizen, D. R. (2013). Updated ultrasound criteria for polycystic ovary syndrome: Reliable thresholds for elevated follicle population and ovarian volume. *Human Reproduction, 28*(5), 1361–1368.

Nilsestuen, L. (2013). IUD perforation to the urinary bladder: Ultrasonographic diagnosis. *Journal of Diagnostic Medical Sonography, 29*(3), 126–129.

Parikh, T., Cruzak, M., Bui, N., Wildner, C., Koch, B., Leko, E., . . . Ellis, S. (2018). Novel use of ultrasound to teach reproductive system physical examination skills and pelvic anatomy. *Journal of Ultrasound in Medicine, 37*, 709–715.

Tsuda, H., Ito, Y. M., Todo, Y., Iba, T., Tasaka, K., Sutou, Y., . . . Yokoyama, Y. Measurement of endometrial thickness in premenopausal women in office gynecology. *Reproductive Medicine and Biology, 17*(1), 29–35. Retrieved from https://www.ncbi.nlm.nih.gov/pmc/articles/PMC5768977

Nowitzki, K., Hoimes, M., Chen, B., Zheng, L., & Kim, Y. (2015). Ultrasonography of intrauterine devices. *Ultrasonography, 34*(3) 183–194. doi: 10.14366/usg.15010

Rosen, M., Shen, S., Dobson, A., Rinaudo, P., McCulloch, C., & Cedars, M. (2008). A quantitative assessment of follicle size on oocyte developmental competence. *Fertility and Sterility, 90*(3), 684–690.

Williams, T., Mortada, R., & Porter, S. (2016). Diagnosis and treatment of polycystic ovarian syndrome. *American Family Physician, 94*(2), 106–113.

Zatel, Y., Sorian, D., Lipitz, S., Mashiach, S., & Achiron, R. (2000). Contribution of color Doppler flow to the ultrasonographic diagnosis of tubal abnormalities. *Journal of Ultrasound in Medicine, 19*(9), 645–649.

CHAPTER 4

Ultrasound in the First Trimester

During the first trimester of pregnancy, clinical situations may warrant a limited or point-of-care (POC) ultrasound examination when a specific piece of information is needed to provide optimal bedside care in a timely fashion. Some of the more common clinical presentations leading to a POC ultrasound examination include vaginal spotting or bleeding, lower abdominal cramping or pain, and the inability of the clinician to auscultate a fetal heart rate (FHR). However, a POC ultrasound is not intended to replace a standard first-trimester ultrasound. If a standard ultrasound study has not been performed prior to the POC imaging, it is recommended that, whenever reasonably possible, the POC scan be followed with a complete standard study (American College of Obstetricians and Gynecologists [ACOG], 2016; American Institute of Ultrasound in Medicine [AIUM], 2018). If critical information is needed when a standard ultrasound is not available, however, a POC ultrasound is certainly a valuable tool for providing timely diagnostic assistance.

The intention of this chapter is to describe each of the components of the standard first-trimester ultrasound examination, from which components may be selected for the POC or limited sonograms. For comparison purposes, some abnormal findings are presented to assist with sonographic distinctions from normal findings, although the detection of fetal anomalies is outside the scope of the majority of advanced practitioners (American College of Nurse Midwives [ACNM], 2016).

▶ Indications for First-Trimester Standard Sonogram

In 1984, the National Institutes of Health (NIH) convened a task force to determine whether routine sonography was appropriate for all pregnancies. Their conclusion at that time was that not all pregnant women would benefit from a routine ultrasound. In turn, a list of appropriate indications warranting sonography was generated for all trimesters of pregnancy (National Institute of Health and Human Development [NICHD], 1984). That basic premise still exists today; however, the indications for a first-trimester ultrasound examination have been updated in recent years (ACOG, 2016) and are shown in **BOX 4-1**. Note that many of the individual indications identified are also indications for a POC ultrasound examination under certain clinical situations.

Confirm the presence of an intrauterine pregnancy

Evaluate a suspected ectopic pregnancy

Define the cause of vaginal bleeding

Evaluate pelvic pain

Estimate gestational age

Diagnose or evaluate multiple gestations

Confirm cardiac activity

Localize and remove an intrauterine device

Assess for certain fetal anomalies

Evaluate maternal pelvic masses or uterine abnormalities

As an adjunct to chorionic villus sampling or embryo transfer

Measure nuchal translucency as part of aneuploidy screening

Evaluate a suspected hydatidiform mole

Modified from ACOG, 2016; AIUM, 2018; NIH, 1984.

▶ Discriminatory Zone in First-Trimester Evaluation

Although management issues are not directly addressed in this text, it is necessary to discuss threatened early pregnancy loss, because a shift in ultrasound interpretation has occurred over the last few years. Serum screening for quantitative beta human chorionic gonadotropin (β-hCG) has been the "gold standard" for many years in assessing the stable patient for an abnormal pregnancy. Although it is not diagnostic, it may be used in conjunction with sonographic evaluation. However, the best approach for patient management will depend on the availability of the testing procedure, the skills of the clinician performing the sonogram, and the interpretation of the results of each.

In the past, certain ranges or cutoffs of β-hCG levels, known as the "discriminatory zone," were used in conjunction with specific first-trimester ultrasound findings to differentiate viable pregnancies from

nonviable pregnancies. Research has shown many drawbacks of that system, and its use is no longer recommended. Doubilet and Benson (2010) determined that two types of errors in image interpretation may potentially lead to errors in management when utilizing this approach: (1) the failure to conclude there is a definite or probable viable pregnancy in conflict with ultrasound images showing such a finding, and (2) the failure to conclude that there is sonographic confirmation or likelihood of the presence of an ectopic pregnancy despite ultrasound images supporting that finding. As a result, ACOG (2018) cautions that "if the hCG discriminatory level is to be used as a diagnostic aid in women at risk of ectopic pregnancy, the value should be conservatively high (e.g., as high as 3,500 mIU/mL) to avoid the potential for misdiagnosis and possible interruption of an intrauterine pregnancy that a woman hopes to continue."

The first potential error may come from failing to see a double sac sign (DSS) or the intradecidual sign (IDS), interpreting the findings as a nonviable pregnancy, and moving forward with medical or surgical intervention. The DSS is thought to represent the two layers of decidua surrounding the intrauterine fluid collection; it appears in most, but not all, normal pregnancies. There are no data to support that the absence of this finding is consistent with an abnormal pregnancy.

The second potential problem is the misdiagnosis of a pseudogestational sac—that is, fluid in the uterine cavity that is occasionally seen in women with an ectopic pregnancy. Fluid in the endometrium is more likely to be a gestational sac than a pseudogestational sac. When nonspecific intrauterine fluid collection is seen, the odds of a gestational sac versus a pseudogestational sac are approximately 245:1. If no intrauterine sac is seen and the patient's quantitative β-hCG is well above a discriminatory level where one expects to see an intrauterine pregnancy (IUP), there should be concern for an ectopic pregnancy. If a sonogram shows a definite extrauterine pregnancy (an embryo with cardiac activity), then the presence or absence of a pseudogestational sac is clinically irrelevant (ACOG, 2016).

Doubilet and Benson (2013) also investigated the interobserver agreement, frequency of occurrence, and prognostic importance of the DSS, the IDS, and other sonographic findings in early pregnancies. In terms of the occurrence of these signs, the interobserver agreement was poor because the sonographic images frequently did not demonstrate either sign. The presence of a DSS or IDS was also unrelated to β-hCG levels, first-trimester outcome, presence of an inner echogenic ring, or decidual presence. The conclusion was that the sonographic appearance of an early gestational sac, before visualization of a yolk sac or embryo, is highly variable. Therefore, if a round or oval intrauterine fluid collection is sonographically visualized in a woman with a positive β-hCG, it should be treated as a gestational sac until proven otherwise, regardless of whether it demonstrates a DSS or an IDS. Performing medical and surgical interventions has the potential to damage an IUP, and these procedures should be avoided unless a viable pregnancy is definitely excluded by follow-up β-hCG values or sonograms (Doubilet & Benson, 2013).

▶ Transvaginal Sonography in the First Trimester

One of the most important prognostic indicators in the first trimester is the crown–rump length (CRL) of the fetus. It is the most accurate biometric measurement for predicting gestational age, and also has predictive value in determining the survivability of a pregnancy (ACOG, 2016; Dutta & Economides, 2003). The development of transvaginal sonography (TVS), along with improved resolution, has led to improved accuracy in CRL measurement. Transvaginal (TV) sonography uses higher-frequency transducers, which provides a 40% to 50% improvement in lateral and axial resolution over transabdominal sonography (TAS). Although AIUM (2018) states that first-trimester ultrasound may be performed by the transabdominal (TA) approach only, most sonographers employ both TV and TA transducers during the standard first-trimester scan.

▶ The Standard Sonographic Exam

Membranes, Yolk Sac, and Umbilical Cord

With a normally developing pregnancy, certain parameters are expected to be visible by TVS at specific gestational ages. The identifiable gestational sac is typically present at 5 weeks' gestation. The yolk sac, located within the chorioamniotic space, becomes visible at 5½ weeks. A small fetal pole can be seen by 6 to 6½ weeks, along with cardiac activity within the pole. The thin and wispy amniotic membrane is sonographically visualized at 7 weeks. As the amniotic cavity grows to the size of the chorion, its expansion obliterates the chorioamniotic space. By 14 to 16 weeks' gestation, the amnion fuses with the chorion, making the two sonographically indistinguishable.

Gestational Sac

Endometrial implantation of the blastocyst occurs approximately 9½ days after conception. Prior to the identification of a normal gestational sac, the endometrium appears secretory. Sonographically, a double-echogenic ring or decidual reaction is produced by the decidual capsularis and the decidua parietalis.

The normal gestational sac can be seen as early as 4 to 5 weeks' gestation or when the sac is 2 to 5 mm in size (Dutta & Economides, 2003). In the past, the gestational sac size has been used to predict gestational age before the identification of the embryo. The normal gestational sac typically appears ellipsoid or circular in shape. Sonographically, it appears as a hypoechoic or anechoic area in or near the midline of the uterus (**FIGURE 4-1**). To obtain the gestational sac size, the sac is measured in all three dimensions at the chorionic margin (**FIGURE 4-2**). One of these planes should be made at the largest diameter of the sac. These measurements are then averaged together.

A mean sac diameter of 25 mm or greater with no visible embryo is diagnostic of a failed pregnancy.

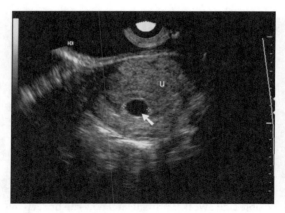

FIGURE 4-1 Transvaginal sonographic image of a normal 6½-week gestational sac (arrow) showing the sac within the uterus (U).

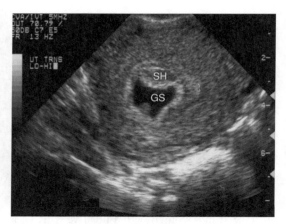

FIGURE 4-3 An irregular gestational sac, as seen in this transvaginal image, has been associated with an abnormal pregnancy. GS = gestational sac, SH = subchorionic hemorrhage.

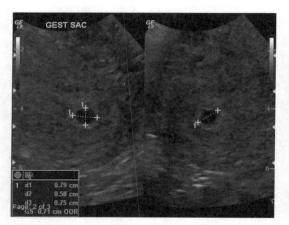

FIGURE 4-2 Gestational sac measurement in two coronal views. The sac is the anechoic area within the uterine cavity. The sac is the anechoic area within the hyperechoic uterine cavity.

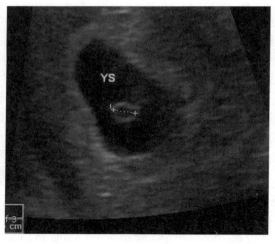

FIGURE 4-4 Gestational sac with presence of yolk sac (YS), noted between measurement cursors.

An abnormal shape to the gestational sac may suggest an abnormal pregnancy (**FIGURE 4-3**); this relationship was first established in 1986 (Nyberg, Laing, & Filly, 1986). Additionally, the gestational sac should increase in size by 1 to 1.2 mm/day. Any abnormal growth of the gestational sac is a poor prognostic sign (ACOG, 2016)

The yolk sac is the next structure that becomes visible, typically between 5 and 6 weeks' gestation. It is located outside the amnion and appears as an echogenic ring with an anechoic center (**FIGURES 4-4 and 4-5**). An irregular yolk sac shape is unrelated to an increased risk of spontaneous abortion (Tan, Pektas, & Arslan, 2012); however, a small yolk sac with a diameter less than 3 mm between 6–10 weeks or a diameter of more than 7 mm before 9 weeks may be suspicious for an abnormal pregnancy and requires a follow-up ultrasound examination to assess pregnancy viability (Abuhamad, 2014).

The yolk sac, fetal pole, and fetal heart can be seen earlier by TV ultrasound than by the TA approach (**TABLE 4-1**). Therefore, if the scan has been performed transabdominally but has not produced evidence of any identifiable fetal anatomy or landmarks, a TV approach should be used.

The Embryo/Fetus

An embryo can first be identified with a TV transducer at approximately 5 to 6 weeks' gestation. Cardiac motion should be observed when the embryo is 2 mm or greater in length. If cardiac activity is not observed when the embryo is greater than 7 mm in length, a subsequent scan 1 week later is recommended to confirm a viable versus a nonviable pregnancy. This should be performed prior to any medical or surgical interventions (ACOG, 2016; AIUM, 2018). The fetal number should be confidently identified beginning at approximately 8 weeks' gestation.

Crown–Rump Length Measurement

Even with extraordinary advances in high-resolution technology, the most accurate method for determining gestational age remains the fetal CRL (**FIGURE 4-6**). In spite of radical improvements in imaging and the ability to date pregnancy accurately (especially with assisted reproductive technologies), there has been minimal improvement in the accuracy of CRL. Accuracy of this early pregnancy ultrasound is measured in terms of a low margin of error, which remains at plus or minus 3 days of the calculated date (ACOG, 2016). As pregnancy advances, this margin of error becomes greater; it will never be as low (or accurate) as it is in the early weeks.

The CRL measures 8 to 14 mm in the sixth week of pregnancy, 14 to 20 mm in the seventh week, and 21 to 30 mm in the eighth week. The early embryo grows approximately 2 mm per day during the first

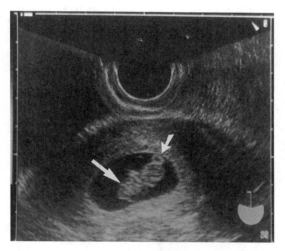

FIGURE 4-5 Yolk sac (at top, smaller arrow) and fetal pole.

TABLE 4-1 Transvaginal Versus Transabdominal Ultrasound: Earliest Visualized Sonographic Findings

Sonographic Finding at Earliest Gestation	Point When Visualized via Transvaginal Scan	Point When Visualized via Transabdominal Scan
Intrauterine sac	4½–5 weeks, measuring 2–4 mm	5½ weeks
Cardiac activity	5 weeks	6 weeks
Yolk sac	5 weeks, measuring 3–5 mm	5½–6 weeks

Modified from ACOG, 2016; AIUM, 2018; Champion, Doubilet, Benson, & Blaivas, 2013.

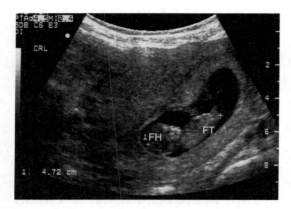

FIGURE 4-6 Transabdominal image of an 11-week, 2-day fetus showing a typical crown–rump length measurement (between cursors). FH = fetal head, FT = fetal torso.

trimester. With few exceptions, the CRL in the normal pregnancy is thought to be biologically stable and, therefore, reproducible and reliable. It usually is not influenced by intrinsic variables such as racial variation or extrinsic variables such as altitude.

Two exceptions to this observation have been demonstrated in one recent study:

- Female embryos showed slightly smaller CRLs than did male embryos.
- Embryos of diabetic mothers had slightly smaller CRLs than did embryos of nondiabetic mothers.

Female fetuses grow considerably more slowly than male fetuses, and these differences are observed from early gestation. However, the female fetus is not merely a smaller version of the male fetus; rather, there is a sex-specific growth pattern for each of the individual fetal biometric indices. These findings provide support for the use of sex-specific sonographic models for fetal weight estimation, as well as the use of sex-specific reference growth charts (Melamed et al., 2013).

Advanced biometry in the first trimester, such as measurement of the biparietal diameter, head circumference, and abdominal circumference, has been studied, and growth charts have been created for the first trimester. The latest research is supportive of greater use of biometry in the first trimester as it potentially allows for more accurate pregnancy dating, enables earlier detection of fetal anomalies

and multiple gestations, and identifies pregnancies at increased risk for aneuploidy (Porche, Warsof, & Abuhamad, 2016). After about 11 or 12 weeks' gestation, the fetal posture may vary between flexion and extension, leading to more variance in the estimated gestational age. The CRL, however, continues to be the most accurate predictor of gestational age.

Fetal Heart Motion

Fetal heart motion can be seen with TV ultrasonography at approximately 5 weeks (CRL of 2–4 mm) in 80% of cases and by 7 weeks in 100% of cases (**FIGURE 4-7**) Cardiac motion is usually seen when the embryo is at least 5 mm in length (ACOG, 2016).

The presence or absence of cardiac activity should be documented with a video clip or M-mode imaging, avoiding use of color or spectral Doppler (ACOG, 2016; AIUM, 2018). When attempting to obtain the FHR with a diagnostic ultrasound system, AIUM recommends using M-mode first because of its lower acoustic intensity. Spectral Doppler has higher acoustic intensity and should not be used. This restriction does not apply to traditional handheld Doppler devices without

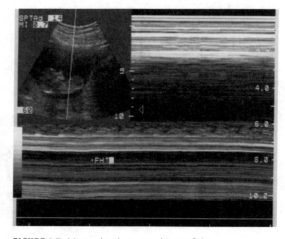

FIGURE 4-7 M-mode ultrasound is useful in documenting fetal heart motion and is the only recommended ultrasound technique for assessing fetal heart rate in the first trimester. M-mode records one-line sonographic information and displays it over time, so that structures that move within that line show a "wavy" pattern on the display.

imaging capabilities that are used to auscultate FHR (AIUM, 2011).

Heart rate may prove to be a useful method of assessing gestational age and predicting impending fetal loss. Fetal loss has been associated not only with the ultrasound finding of a small gestational sac, but also with fetal bradycardia (less than 90–100 bpm) (Yi et al., 2016).

Fetal Structural Abnormalities

Many fetal structural abnormalities can be identified as early as the first trimester (**FIGURE 4-8**). A limited anatomic survey can be accomplished as early as 12 weeks' gestation, although not all anomalies can be identified at this point (Harper, Wood, Jenkins, Owen, & Biggio, 2016). Anomalies can occur either as isolated findings or as part of a syndrome. Although a variety of defects have been identified in early pregnancy, an abnormal nuchal translucency (NT) is the most reliable finding. As stated by the Fetal Medicine Foundation (FMF, 2018), "screening by NT can detect about 80% of fetuses with trisomy 21 and other major aneuploides for a false positive rate of 5%."

Nuchal Translucency

The "prominent nuchal membrane" was first described in 1990 by Szabo and Gellen, and is now referred to as *nuchal translucency* (FMF, 2018; Taipale, Ammala, Salonen, & Hiilesmaa, 2003). Nuchal translucency is an abnormal collection of fluid in the posterior cervical (nuchal) area of the fetus that can be detected as early as 9 weeks' gestation. These fluid accumulations have been described as localized or diffuse, thick or septated, transient or permanent collections of fluid, and are associated with an increased incidence of chromosomal anomalies (FMF, 2018) (**FIGURES 4-9** and **4-10**).

Normal nuchal *thickening* (as opposed to translucency) increases with gestational age. Therefore, it is recommended that the NT measurement be performed between 10 and 13 weeks' gestation, with a cutoff measurement typically being less than 3 mm and dependent on CRL. With a measurement of more than 3 mm, there is a 10% increase in major congenital anomalies. Originally, research had shown the risk of anomaly increased to 90% with a measurement of 6 mm (Smith & Smith, 2003); however, it was found that using NT measurement alone produced a high degree of false positives. At this point in time, more detailed calculations are done, taking into consideration the maternal age, fetal heart rate, and maternal serum free ß-hCG and Pappalysin-1 (PAPP-A) along with the fetal nuchal translucency measurement (FMF, 2018).

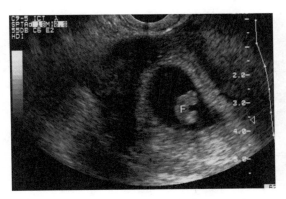

FIGURE 4-8 This fetus (F) was found to be anomalous at the time of this 9-week ultrasound examination. Although a heartbeat could be seen, no normal fetal anatomy could be visualized.

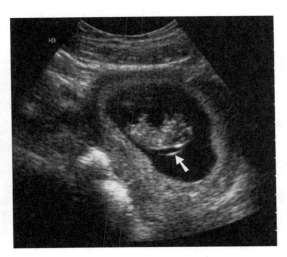

FIGURE 4-9 Increased nuchal translucency (arrow) was determined during ultrasound examination of this 11-week fetus with trisomy 21.

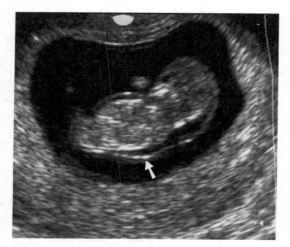

FIGURE 4-10 In addition to the nuchal translucency, this fetus has diffused anasarca (widespread edema) pushing skin away from the torso (arrow). Chorionic villus sampling showed this fetus to have monosomy X (Turner's syndrome).

An extended fetal neck can result in a falsely increased measurement. Additionally, careful attention needs to be given to the placement of the calipers when obtaining the measurement so as to avoid mistaking the amnion, a spinal defect, or encephalocele for nuchal thickening (FMF, 2018). The nuchal region should be assessed during the first-trimester sonogram. The resulting measurement should be used in conjunction with biochemical markers to determine the risk for aneuploidy and other abnormalities. The measurements must be done at a precise level by an experienced practitioner to ensure the accuracy of the result (ACOG, 2016; AIUM, 2018). Advanced practitioners who are interested in incorporating NT measurements into their ultrasound practice are encouraged to attain certification (FMF, 2018).

Adnexa and Uterus

The complete first-trimester sonographic examination should include an assessment of the myometrium and the adnexa (ACOG, 2016). Evaluation of the adnexa can include both TA and TV ultrasound examinations. The depth of penetration of the TV sound beam is restricted due to its high frequency and can restrict visualization of the deep adnexa. As a result, large masses, such as those extending from the uterine fundus, can missed. In these situations, a TA ultrasound examination should also be performed. In addition, the uterus and the adnexa should be evaluated for masses and evidence of an extrauterine gestation. The cul-de-sac should be evaluated for the presence or absence of fluid (ACOG, 2016; AIUM, 2018).

The normal myometrium should have a uniformly homogenous, echogenic appearance. By comparison, the peritoneum (perimetrium) and endometrium are stronger reflectors and appear more echogenic by ultrasound. Uterine masses, such as leiomyomata, may present as discrete entities in the myometrial substance, or they may appear as diffuse thickening of the myometrium. Commonly, the diffuse thickening is adenomyosis rather than a fibroid, with true fibroids having definitive borders. Submucosal leiomyomata or polyps in the endometrial cavity may distort the usual linear appearance of the endometrial echo (**FIGURE 4-11**). Pedunculated leiomyomata that extend into the adnexa can mimic solid or complex adnexal masses.

Both ovaries should also be investigated during the first-trimester standard scan. A corpus luteal cyst of pregnancy is a common adnexal finding in the first trimester. It is usually unilateral and can appear anechoic or complex. It may become hemorrhagic, resulting in an echo-filled texture on the image, or it may develop thick walls. The corpus luteal cyst

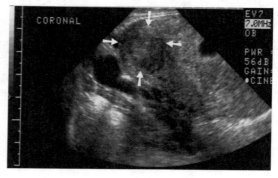

FIGURE 4-11 Uterine leiomyomata (arrows), such as this one seen on a transabdominal sonographic image, are common and often are observed during routine examination.

typically resolves by 16 weeks' gestation. Rarely, such a cyst may grossly enlarge, becoming symptomatic and measuring more than 10 cm.

The components of the standard first-trimester obstetric sonogram are summarized in **BOX 4-2**.

▶ Sonography in Early Pregnancy Complications

Threatened Abortion

The two most common indications for a first-trimester sonogram are vaginal bleeding or spotting and abdominal or pelvic pain, both of which may be indicative of a threatened abortion. When used appropriately, POC sonography can be used confidently to distinguish the normal IUP from such pathologic conditions as missed and spontaneous abortion, ectopic pregnancy, or hydatidiform mole.

As mentioned earlier, the identification of various sonographic landmarks, such as detection of heart motion or a yolk sac, has served to predict successful pregnancy continuation. In addition, much effort has been applied to finding biochemical and sonographic parameters with prognostic capabilities in cases of threatened abortion. Along this line, another ultrasound prognostic sign, subchorionic hemorrhage (SCH), has been described (Figure 4-3). This finding is characterized by a hypoechoic collection of fluid outside the gestational sac. It has been associated with miscarriage and preterm labor, but in most cases is an insignificant finding (Deutchman, Tubay, & Turok, 2009; Yamada et al., 2012). Although SCH increases the risk of miscarriage, it does not appear to be an absolute predictor of impending loss (Şükür et al., 2014).

Anembryonic Gestation or Nonliving Embryo/Fetus

An anembryonic pregnancy, previously referred to as a blighted ovum, usually represents an early IUP failure with subsequent embryonic disintegration. This gives the appearance of an "empty sac." The anembryonic pregnancy can be diagnosed confidently when the mean gestational sac size is greater than 25 mm with no embryo identified (ACOG, 2016; Champion et al., 2013). TVS, however, has allowed for an earlier confident diagnosis. Once a mean gestational sac diameter of 10 mm is achieved, a yolk sac should be identifiable. If a yolk sac cannot be seen at this time, an anembryonic pregnancy may be diagnosed (**FIGURE 4-12**).

Missed Abortion

The missed abortion has been defined as an intrauterine embryo with a CRL of greater than 15 mm without fetal cardiac motion. Sonographically, these fetuses can be hydropic, with diffuse edema (Figure 4-10) (Tan et al., 2012).

Pregnancy of Unknown Location

If during either a POC sonogram or a standard first-trimester ultrasound examination, the location of the pregnancy cannot be definitively determined, the diagnosis may be a pregnancy of

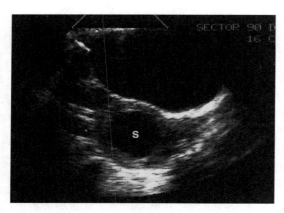

FIGURE 4-12 Sagittal transabdominal image showing an anembryonic (blighted ovum) gestational sac (S).

unknown location (PUL). Barnhart and associates (2011) have proposed a consensus statement with definitions of population, target disease, and final outcome in such cases:

- *Definite extrauterine pregnancy (EP):* Extrauterine gestational sac with yolk sac and/or embryo (with or without cardiac activity)
- *Probable EP:* Homogeneous adnexal mass or extrauterine sac-like structure
- *PUL:* No signs of either EP or IUP
- *Probable IUP:* Intrauterine echogenic sac-like structure
- *Definite IUP:* Intrauterine gestational sac with yolk sac and/or embryo (with or without cardiac activity)

Ectopic Pregnancy

In addition to tools such as serum quantitative β-hCG levels and physical examination, sonography plays a pivotal role in the diagnosis and management of ectopic pregnancy. The most widely accepted diagnostic application of sonography in a suspected ectopic pregnancy is the lack of identification of an IUP in the presence of sufficiently high serum quantitative β-hCG levels that would normally be seen with an IUP. Conversely, the presence of an IUP or yolk sac virtually excludes the possibility of an ectopic pregnancy, except for the risk of a

heterotopic pregnancy (one twin intrauterine and one twin extrauterine). The risk of heterotopic pregnancy is 1/30,000 for spontaneous conceptions and 1/6000 in assisted reproduction conceptions (Goettler, & Zanetti-Dällenbach, 2016; Hill, 2003).

Ultrasound findings of an ectopic pregnancy may include an empty uterus with or without a thickened endometrium, a pseudogestational sac in the uterus, a concurrent intrauterine (heterotopic) pregnancy, or the absence of a gestational sac at 6 weeks' gestation (**FIGURES 4-13** and **4-14**). In approximately 10% to 20% of ectopic pregnancies, a gestational sac can be seen outside the endometrial cavity with an identifiable embryonic/fetal pole and an active heartbeat. This finding provides convincing evidence of an ectopic pregnancy. More commonly, findings of a noncystic adnexal mass or fluid (simple or complex) in the posterior cul-de-sac are observed with the ectopic pregnancy.

Trophoblastic Disease and Placental Issues

Trophoblastic disease, or molar pregnancy, is a rare complication of pregnancy that may present as vaginal bleeding. It results from a degeneration of placental tissue. The incidence of trophoblastic disease varies widely throughout the world, with

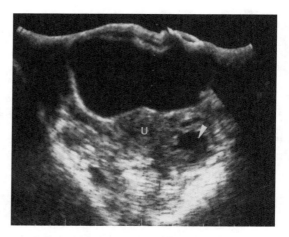

FIGURE 4-13 Transverse image of ectopic pregnancy (arrowhead) and uterus (U).

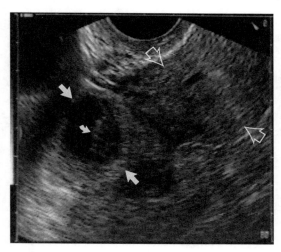

FIGURE 4-14 Transvaginal image of a right adnexal ectopic pregnancy with a gestational sac (large arrows) and fetal pole (small arrow). The uterus is seen (hollow arrows) with a small amount of endometrial fluid.

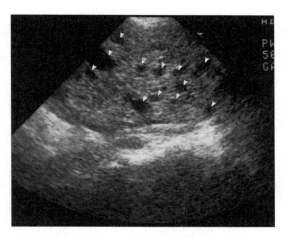

FIGURE 4-15 Gestational trophoblastic disease: Real-time image of the uterus reveals a soft-tissue mass with multiple cystic areas (arrowheads) of varying sizes, often described as a grape-like pattern.

reported ranges from 12/1000 pregnancies in Indonesia, India, and Turkey to 0.5/1000 pregnancies in North America and Europe (Shaaban et al., 2017). There are basically two types: a complete mole, in which there is no embryonic tissue (**FIGURE 4-15**), and an incomplete mole, in which the embryo

develops in the presence of a hydropic placenta. Sonographically, a molar pregnancy may appear as a "grape-like" cluster in the intrauterine cavity.

Morbidly Adherent Placenta

Another placental concern that may raise suspicion in the first trimester is the morbidly adherent placenta (MAP; inclusive of accreta, increta, or percreta). The incidence of MAP occurring in women with prior uterine incisions is now 1 in every 500 births (Turan, 2017). Sonographic findings of a potential MAP in the first trimester include women with persistent placenta previa or low-lying placenta who also show the smallest anterior myometrial thickness, thus improving the ability to predict a developing morbidly adherent placenta (Rac et al., 2016). Although this exam is not within the scope of practice of the vast majority of advanced practice clinicians, should the cesarean birth rate continue to rise, the incidence of this extremely severe placental complication may also continue to rise. Earlier identification than is possible now may have an impact on future treatment modalities, thereby affecting maternal morbidity and mortality.

▶ Summary

Advances in reproductive technologies and medical therapies have contributed to higher pregnancy rates and, in turn, to higher rates of complications in the first trimester. Physical, biochemical, and sonographic assessments are intimately interwoven in the evaluation of patients with early pregnancy complications. Clinically relevant and realistic goals of sonography in the first trimester include (1) visualization and localization of the gestational sac and the exclusion of an ectopic pregnancy, (2) early identification of nonviable pregnancies, (3) determination of the number of embryos, (4) estimation of gestational age, and (5) early diagnosis of fetal abnormalities. High-resolution vaginal ultrasound has greatly enhanced the clinician's ability to assess the pregnancy. Additionally, in the stable woman with an inconclusive sonogram, subsequent repeat sonogram(s) may improve the accuracy of diagnosis. A completely empty uterus, even without evidence of endometrial fluid collection, and a β-hCG level of greater than 2000 mIU/mL does not exclude the development of a normal IUP (Doubilet, 2013).

POC ultrasound in the first trimester offers many advantages in patient care. Notably, it can eliminate delays in diagnosis, management, and treatment. By doing so, it also improves patient safety and satisfaction. However, performing a more limited ultrasound examination instead of a standard sonogram carries some inherent risks. A general rule of thumb is that if something is not visualized when it is expected to be seen, or if the pregnancy is not clearly identified in the uterus, a standard ultrasound examination is indicated before any medical or surgical interventions can be carried out to ensure that a viable but misdated pregnancy is not interrupted.

Study Questions

1. Is there any predictive value that can be attributed to the presence/absence of the double sac sign?
    a. Nearly 100% of normal pregnancies have a double sac sign.
    b. There are no data to support that the absence of this finding is consistent with an abnormal pregnancy.
    c. Approximately 25% of abnormal pregnancies have a double sac sign.

2. What is the fluid visualized in the endometrial cavity during the first trimester most likely to represent?
    a. A gestational sac
    b. A pseudogestational sac
    c. An empty sac

3. If a round or oval intrauterine fluid collection is sonographically visualized in a woman with a positive β-hCG, how should it be treated?
    a. As a pseudogestational sac until proven otherwise
    b. As an empty sac signifying a anembryonic pregnancy
    c. As a gestational sac until proven otherwise

4. What is the most important prognostic indicator for the crown–rump length in the first trimester?
    a. Determination of the survivability of a pregnancy
    b. Determination of fetal structural anomalies
    c. Estimated gestational age

5. Which major improvement did the development of transvaginal sonography provide in regard to sonography?
    a. Earlier detection of anembryonic pregnancies
    b. Improvement in lateral and axial resolution over transabdominal sonography
    c. Lower power output, and, therefore, lower incidence of potential fetal effects

6. At what gestational age should the gestational sac typically be visible with TVS?
    a. 5 weeks
    b. 6 weeks
    c. 7 weeks

7. When does the amnion fuse with the chorion, making the two sonographically indistinguishable?
    a. 6–8 weeks' gestation
    b. 14–16 weeks' gestation
    c. 20–22 weeks' gestation

8. How does the gestational sac sonographically appear in the first trimester?
    a. As an hypoechoic or anechoic area anywhere within the uterine cavity
    b. As an hyperechoic area in or near the midline of the uterus
    c. As an hypoechoic or anechoic area in or near the midline of the uterus

9. What size will the normal gestation sac be at 4 to 5 weeks' gestation?
    a. 2–5 mm
    b. 6–10 mm
    c. 11–14 mm

10. How does the normal gestational sac typically appear in the first trimester?
    a. Ellipsoid or circular in shape
    b. Only circular
    c. Only ellipsoid

11. How is the gestational sac size is obtained?
    a. By averaging the measurements obtained in two dimensions at the chorionic margin
    b. By measuring the largest dimension only at the largest portion at the chorionic margin
    c. By averaging the measurements obtained in three dimensions at the chorionic margin

12. What sac diameter with no visible embryo is diagnostic of an anembryonic pregnancy?
    a. 20 mm
    b. 25 mm
    c. 30 mm

13. How does an irregular yolk sac shape relate to the risk of spontaneous pregnancy loss?
    a. It is unrelated to an increased risk.
    b. The risk is doubled.
    c. The risk is unknown.

14. When an embryo can first be identified with a TV transducer?
    a. At approximately 5 to 6 weeks' gestation
    b. At approximately 4 to 5 weeks' gestation
    c. Definitely by 5 weeks' gestation

15. By what embryonic measurement should cardiac motion should be observed?
    a. More than 4 mm in length
    b. More than 6 mm in length
    c. More than 2 mm in length

16. If cardiac activity is not observed when it is expected, what should the management include?
    a. Consultation regarding uterine evacuation for nonviable pregnancy
    b. Offering medical management for the nonviable pregnancy
    c. Repeat ultrasound in 1 week before concluding it is a nonviable pregnancy

17. At what gestational age should an experienced sonographer be able to confidently and accurately determine fetal number following ovarian stimulation?
    a. 6–8 weeks
    b. 8–10 weeks
    c. 10–12 weeks

18. What are the earliest gestational age and fetal length at which cardiac motion should be visualized in 80% of fetuses when TV ultrasound is used?
    a. Fetal heart motion at approximately 5 weeks and a CRL of 2–4 mm
    b. Fetal heart motion at approximately 7 weeks and a CRL of 6–8 mm
    c. Fetal heart motion at approximately 9 weeks and a CRL of 10–12 mm

19. If the presence or absence of cardiac activity cannot be documented with the transvaginal probe, what would the next step be?
    a. Turn on color flow Doppler
    b. Use M-mode imaging
    c. Use spectral Doppler

20. Which ultrasound findings have a strong association with fetal loss?
    a. Small gestational sac and/or fetal bradycardia (less than 90–100 bpm)
    b. Large gestation sac and/or fetal tachycardia (more than 160–180 bpm)
    c. Normal size gestational sac and/or fetal bradycardia (less than 100–120 bpm)

21. What is the recommended time frame for when NT measurement may be performed?
    a. Between 18 and 20 weeks' gestation
    b. Between 14 and 16 weeks' gestation
    c. Between 10 and 13 weeks' gestation

22. What is the rationale for using both TA and TV ultrasound when evaluating the adnexa?
    a. The depth of penetration of the TV sound beam is restricted due to its high frequency and can limit visualization of the deep adnexa.
    b. The pregnant uterus can obliterate the visualization of the adnexa when using a transabdominal transducer.
    c. The depth of penetration of the TV transducer allows for accurate and detailed assessment of the adnexa because it is closer to the structures.

23. How is a subchorionic hemorrhage sonographically described?
    a. A hyperechoic collection of fluid inside the gestational sac
    b. A hypoechoic collection of fluid outside the gestational sac
    c. A hyperechoic collection of fluid outside the gestational sac

24. Which pregnancy outcome can be anticipated with a subchorionic hemorrhage?
    a. It has been associated with miscarriage and preterm labor, but in most cases is an insignificant finding.
    b. It has been associated with pregnancy loss in most cases.
    c. It is considered an insignificant finding requiring no intervention.

25. How is a missed abortion sonographically diagnosed?
    a. A gestational sac larger than 25 mm with no embryo
    b. An embryo with a CRL of greater than 15 mm without fetal cardiac motion
    c. An embryo with a CRL of greater than 25 mm without fetal cardiac motion

26. With TVS, once a mean gestational sac diameter of 10 mm is achieved, what else should be seen in a normal pregnancy?
    a. A yolk sac should be identifiable.
    b. The chorion and amnion should be fused.
    c. The double decidual sign should be evident.

27. The presence of an IUP or yolk sac virtually excludes the possibility of an ectopic pregnancy, except under which circumstance?
    a. The possibility of a heterozygous twin
    b. Following the use of follicular stimulants
    c. The presence of a heterotopic pregnancy

28. Which of the following is a possible ultrasound finding with an ectopic pregnancy?
    a. An empty uterus with or without a thickened endometrium
    b. The absence of a fetus in a gestational sac larger than 25 mm at 6 weeks' gestation
    c. A grape-like cluster in the intrauterine cavity

29. If the sonographic findings in the first trimester for a woman with a history of prior cesarean section include a persistent placenta previa or low-lying placenta, the appropriate follow-up would include:
    a. a repeat ultrasound in 1 week for placental location.
    b. a repeat ultrasound observing for anterior myometrial thickness.
    c. a repeat ultrasound in the third trimester to determine the placenta/cervical relationship.

30. What cannot be excluded with the following information: completely empty uterus, without evidence of endometrial fluid collection, and with a β-hCG level of greater than 2000 mIU/mL?
    a. A normal pregnancy
    b. An ectopic pregnancy
    c. A trophoblastic molar pregnancy

References

Abuhamad, A. (Ed). (2014). Ultrasound in obstetrics and gynecology: A practical approach. Norfolk, VA: Author.

American College of Obstetricians and Gynecologists (ACOG). (2016). *Ultrasonography in pregnancy. Technical Bulletin No. 175*. Washington, DC: Author.

American College of Obstetricians and Gynecologists (ACOG). (2018). Tubal ectopic pregnancy. Retrieved from https://www.acog.org/Clinical-Guidance-and-Publications/Practice-Bulletins/Committee-on-Practice-Bulletins-Gynecology/Tubal-Ectopic-Pregnancy

American Institute of Ultrasound in Medicine (AIUM). (2011). *AIUM statement on measurement of fetal heart rate*. Laurel, MD: Author.

AIUM-ARC-ACOG-SMFM-SRU (2018). *Practice parameters for the performance of the standard diagnostic obstetric ultrasound examination*. Retrieved from https://www.aium.org/resources/guidelines/obstetric.pdf

Barnhart, K., van Mello, N. M., Bourne, T., Kirk, E., Van Calster, B., Bottomley, C., . . . Timmerman, D. (2011). Pregnancy of unknown location: A consensus statement of nomenclature, definitions, and outcome. *Fertility and Sterility, 95*(3), 857–866.

Champion, E., Doubilet, P., Benson, C., & Blaivas, M. (2013). Current concepts: Diagnostic criteria for nonviable pregnancy early in the first trimester. *New England Journal of Medicine, 369*, 1443–1451.

Deutchman, M., Tubay, A. T., & Turok, D. (2009). First trimester bleeding. *American Family Physician, 79*(11), 985–992.

Doubilet, P. M., & Benson, C. B. (2010). First, do no harm . . . to early pregnancies. *Journal of Ultrasound in Medicine, 29,* 685–689.

Doubilet, P. M., & Benson, C. B. (2013). Double sac sign and intradecidual sign in early pregnancy. *Journal of Ultrasound in Medicine, 32,* 1207–1214.

Dutta, R. L., & Economides, D. L. (2003). Patient acceptance of transvaginal sonography in the early pregnancy unit setting. *Ultrasound in Obstetrics & Gynecology, 22*(5), 503–507.

Fetal Medicine Foundation (FMF). (2018). Nuchal translucency scan. Retrieved from https://fetalmedicine.org/nuchal-translucency-scan

Goettler, S., & Zanetti-Dällenbach, R. (2016). Heterotopic pregnancy. *New England Journal of Medicine, 375,* 1982. doi: 10.1056/NEJMicm1509537.

Harper, L., Wood, S. L., Jenkins, S., Owen, J., & Biggio, J. R. (2016). The performance of first trimester anatomy scan: A decision analysis. *American Journal of Perinatology, 33*(10), 957–965. doi: 10.1055/s-0036-1579652

Hill, J. (2003). Assisted reproduction and the multiple pregnancy: Increasing the risks for heterotopic pregnancy. *Journal of Diagnostic Medical Sonography, 19,* 28–260.

Melamed, N., Meisner, I., Mashiach, R., Wiznitzer, A., Glezerman, M., & Yogev, Y. (2013). Fetal sex and intrauterine growth patterns. *Journal of Ultrasound in Medicine, 32,* 35–43.

National Institutes of Health (NIH). (1984). *Diagnostic ultrasound in pregnancy.* NIH Publication No. 84-667. Bethesda, MD: U.S. Department of Health and Human Services.

Nyberg, D. A., Laing, F. C., & Filly, R. A. (1986). Threatened abortion: Sonographic distinction of normal and abnormal gestation sacs. *Radiology, 158,* 397.

Porche, L. M., Warsof, S., & Abuhamad, A. (2016). Fetal biometry in early pregnancy. In Abramowicz, J. (Ed.), *First-trimester ultrasound* (pp. 153–165). Cham, Switzerland: Springer. doi: https://doi.org/10.1007/978-3-319-20203-7_9

Rac, M., Moschos, E., Wells, C. E., McIntire, D. D., Dashe, J., & Twickler, D. (2016). Sonographic findings of morbidly adherent placenta in the first trimester. *Journal of Ultrasound in Medicine, 35,* 263–269.

Shaaban, A. M., Rezvani, M., Haroun, R. R., Kennedy, A. M., Elsayes, K. M., Olpin, J. D., . . . Menias, C. O. (2017). Gestational trophoblastic disease: Clinical and imaging features. *RadioGraphics, 37*(2). Retrieved from https://doi.org/10.1148/rg.2017160140

Smith, N. C., & Smith, P. M. (2003). *Obstetric ultrasound made easy.* Edinburgh, UK: Churchill Livingstone.

Şükür, Y. E., Göç, G., Köse, O., Açmaz, G., Özmen, B., Atabekoğlu, C. S., Koç, A., & Söylemez, F. (2014). The effects of subchorionic hematoma on pregnancy outcome in patients with threatened abortion. *Journal of the Turkish German Gynecological Association, 15*(4), 239–242. doi: 10.5152/jtgga.2014.14170

Szabo, J., & Gellen, I. (1990). Nuchal fluid accumulation in trisomy 21 detected by vaginosonography in first trimester [Letter]. *Lancet, 336,* 1133.

Taipale, P., Ammala, M., Salonen, R., & Hiilesmaa, V. (2003). Learning curve in ultrasonographic screening for selected fetal structural anomalies in early pregnancy. *Obstetrics and Gynecology, 101*(2), 273–278.

Tan, S., Pektas, M. K., & Arslan, H. (2012). Sonographic evaluation of the yolk sac. *Journal of Ultrasound in Medicine, 31,* 87–95.

Turan, M. (2017). Morbidly adherent placenta: A multi-disciplinary approach. Retrieved from https://www.mdedge.com/obgynnews/article/150150/obstetrics/morbidly-adherent-placenta-multidisciplinary-approach

Yamada, T., Atsuki, Y., Wakasaya, A., Kobayashi, M., Hirano, Y., & Ohwada, M. (2012). Characteristics of patients with subchorionic hematomas in the second trimester. *Journal of Obstetrics and Gynaecology Research, 38*(1), 180–184.

Yi, Y., Lu, G., Ouyang, Y., Gin, G., Gong, F., & Li, X. (2016). A logistic model to predict early pregnancy loss following in vitro fertilization based on 2601 infertility patients. *Reproductive Biology and Endocrinology, 14,* 15. doi: 10.1186/s12958-016-0147-z

CHAPTER 5

Ultrasound in the Second and Third Trimesters

▶ Introduction

Assessment of symptoms and pregnancy complications in the second and third trimesters can be expedited and decision making improved by utilizing sonography in the evaluation of both maternal and fetal conditions. Some of the most common maternal symptoms include bleeding and pain, both of which warrant the use of point-of-care (POC) ultrasound at the bedside because timely results can yield improved outcome.

Another situation in which a POC ultrasound exam is indicated is when a woman who has not had prenatal care presents with signs and symptoms of labor. It may be imperative to determine fetal gestational age and weight, should the delivery be imminent or transfer to another facility indicated. Knowing the approximate sonographic fetal gestational age may assist in determining the need for tocolytics, steroid administration, and neonatal interventions and, therefore, may also impact the long-term outcome. If the birth does not occur as anticipated, then a standard sonogram should be performed as soon as possible.

This chapter describes the components of a standard second- and third-trimester obstetric examination, most elements of which apply to POC ultrasound examinations. Additionally, this chapter contains sample images of deviations-from-normal fetal anatomy that can be used as a basis for comparison with normal fetal anatomic images, with the intention of making the identification of normal anatomic structures easier. Although it is not within the scope of ultrasound practice for most advanced practitioners (APs) to identify fetal anomalies, it is within the scope of practice to recognize normal anatomy, specifically those structures used in biometry.

▶ Indications for Second- and Third-Trimester Standard Scans

Because ultrasound allows for prompt, efficient, and informative decision making, there are numerous indications for performing a second- and/or third-trimester standard scan (**TABLE 5-1**). If a routine ultrasound has not been performed in the first trimester, a fetal anatomic survey may be offered at 18 to 20 weeks' gestation (American College of

TABLE 5-1 Examples of Indications for Second- and Third-Trimester Standard Ultrasound Examination

Estimation of gestational age and weight	Suspected ectopic pregnancy
Evaluation of fetal growth	Rule out fetal demise
Evaluation of fetal well-being	Suspected uterine anomaly
Assessment of amniotic fluid	Suspected placental abruption
Vaginal bleeding	Adjunct to external cephalic version
Cervical insufficiency	Premature rupture of membranes (PROM)
Adjunct to cerclage placement	Abnormal biochemical markers
Determination of presenting part	Follow-up evaluation of fetal anomaly
Fetal number	Follow-up of placental location
Adjunct to amniocentesis or other procedure	History of prior infant with anomaly
Size/dates discrepancy	Assess for indicators for risk of aneuploidy
Pelvic mass	Screening for fetal anomalies
Suspected hydatidiform mole	Abdominal or pelvic pain

Modified from AIUM (2018) and Reddy (2014)

Obstetricians and Gynecologists [ACOG], 2016b, Reddy, Abuhamad, Levine, & Saade, 2014), which is still within the range of securing reasonable gestational dating.

▶ Standard Second- and Third-Trimester Examination

The standard ultrasound performed in the second and third trimesters entails a complete survey, which includes the following elements:

- Taking fetal biometric measurements
- Evaluating specific fetal anatomy
- Identifying the presence or absence of fetal cardiac activity
- Identifying the fetal number (e.g., twins)
- Determining fetal presentation
- Identifying placental localization
- Quantifying the amniotic fluid volume

Additionally, when technically feasible, the maternal cervix and adnexa should be examined based on clinical indicators (Table 5-1) (ACOG, 2016a; American College of Radiology [ACR], 2007; American

Institute of Ultrasound in Medicine [AIUM], 2018, Reddy et al., 2014). Some measurements are used more frequently than others.

Fetal Biometry

Fetal biometry is the sonographic method of obtaining four specific fetal measurements and comparing these findings to standardized estimated fetal weight (EFW) and estimated gestational age (EGA) tables. The individual anatomic measurement or combinations of anatomic measurements will correspond to ranges of fetal weights and gestational ages. The accuracy in estimating fetal weight and gestational age is diminished if only one anatomic measurement is used. The correlations pertaining to the measurements were established decades ago (Hadlock & Deter, 1982; Hadlock, Deter, Harrist, & Park, 1982a, 1982b; Hadlock, Harrist, Deter, & Park, 1982), but are still used in the second and third trimesters of pregnancy today. They include the following:

- Fetal head biparietal diameter (BPD)
- Fetal head circumference (HC)
- Fetal femur length (FL)
- Fetal abdominal circumference (AC)

The gestational age of a pregnancy should never be assigned a new due date based on a second- or third-trimester sonogram *if* a first trimester dating ultrasound has already been performed (ACOG, 2016b). Recalculating the gestational age of a pregnancy at this late point increases the risk of missing a fetal growth disorder. For example, if the third-trimester fetal growth scan indicates a gestational age of 3 weeks less than the gestational age determined by sonogram in the first trimester, that discrepancy in "dating" more accurately indicates a growth-restricted fetus. This type of error can contribute to poor fetal outcome.

Fetal Biparietal Diameter

The BPD is one of the four most common measurements used to determine fetal age. It can be accurately measured after week 12 of the pregnancy. The proper sonographic image is obtained in a transverse view of the head. The correct level is identified when the thalami and the cavum septum pellucidi are visualized and the cerebellar hemispheres are not visible (ACOG, 2016b; AIUM, 2018).

The measurement is obtained by placing a caliper on the proximal or outside edge of the skull nearest the transducer and the second caliper on the inside of the distal skull. This dimension is referred to as the outer-to-inner skull measurement or leading edge-to-leading edge (**FIGURE 5-1**). The inside distal edge of the skull is used because the farther the sound waves travel, the greater the likelihood of creating artifact or a thicker-appearing skull. If the outer edge of the distal skull is used, the BPD (and thus the gestational age) will erroneously be determined to be larger, with an incorrectly advanced gestational age and higher weight. Once the BPD is determined, the software in the ultrasound machine will calculate the EGA and EFW and store it until the remaining measurements have been completed.

These measurements and estimations of gestational age are also based on the fetal head being more oval in shape. Other, less common head shapes include a rounder appearance, known as brachycephalic, and an elongated shape, known as dolichocephalic; these shapes may cause the BPD measurement to be misleading (ACOG, 2016b; AIUM, 2018). Under such circumstances, the head circumference is more accurate than the BPD.

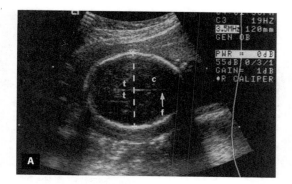

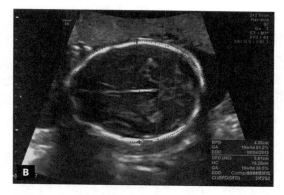

FIGURE 5-1 A. Biparietal diameter (BPD): t, on each side of the thalami; c, over the cavum septi pellucidi; f, at the arrow is the falx cerebri, an echogenic line from anterior to posterior in the cranium. The first caliper is placed on the proximal or outside edge of the skull nearest the transducer and the second caliper on the inside of the distal skull. **B.** BPD on vertical axis. Note the caliper placement. The ellipse indicates head circumference.

Head Circumference

Due to the variations in head shape, measurement of the HC is utilized in determining the EGA and EFW. The HC is considered more precise in determining fetal age because the measurement is not shape dependent (AIUM, 2018). As with the BPD, the HC can be measured after 12 weeks. The HC is obtained in the same view as the BPD, and an ellipse is used to encircle the head (**FIGURES 5-1B** and **5-2**).

A method used less frequently in clinical practice that is not part of routine biometry is the cephalic index (CI). The CI equals the BPD divided

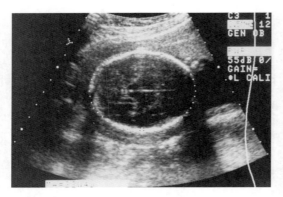

FIGURE 5-2 Head circumference (ellipse encircling the skull at the level of the BPD).

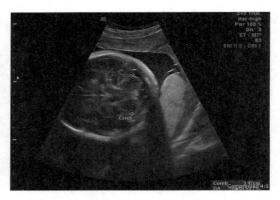

FIGURE 5-4 View and measurement of the cerebellum.

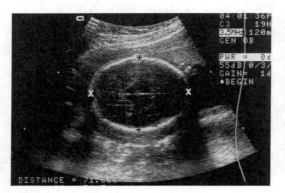

FIGURE 5-3 Cephalic index. It is equal to the BPD (measured from + to +) divided by the occipital–frontal diameter (from × to ×) multiplied by 100.

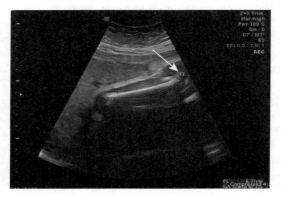

FIGURE 5-5 Hyperechoic femur, with correct placement of cursors (at each end) for measuring femur length. The epiphyses (arrow) are excluded from the measurement.

by the occipital–frontal diameter multiplied by 100 (**FIGURE 5-3**). The CI is an indicator of head shape that is used in the sonographic literature.

When measuring the BPD and HC, the cerebellum should not be visible. If the cerebellum is visible, the scanning plane is too low (**FIGURE 5-4**).

Fetal Femur Length

The FL measurement is used in assessing fetal growth. This measurement is optimal at 15 weeks and remains accurate until approximately 32 weeks. The femur is measured in a longitudinal position. The proper view is obtained when the longest measurement of femur is visualized. The diaphysis of the femur

is echogenic and can display posterior shadowing depending on the gestational age.

The measurement is performed by placing a caliper at each end of the diaphysis, excluding the epiphysis. The epiphysis is hypoechoic, becoming hyperechoic after 32 weeks' gestation (**FIGURE 5-5**). For the best resolution and most accurate measurement, the femur closest to the transducer should be measured. After 32 weeks' gestation, or if the posterior (deep) femur is being measured, the femur may erroneously appear bowed (ACR, 2007). True abnormal bowing may be seen in fetuses with skeletal abnormalities such as hypomineralization or osteogenesis imperfecta, which can lead to bone fractures (**FIGURE 5-6**). Thus, accuracy in technique is imperative to avoid misdiagnosis.

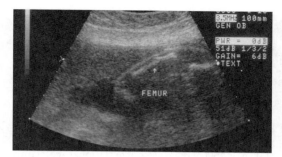

FIGURE 5-6 Femur with hypomineralization. Note the break in the femur at the arrow.

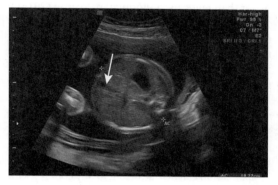

FIGURE 5-7 Abdominal circumference. Arrow indicates portal vein.

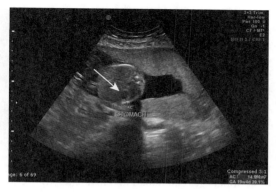

FIGURE 5-8 Transverse image of level for abdominal circumference. AC, abdominal circumference. Note the anechoic stomach bubble (arrow).

The FL measurement is calculated for gestational age by the ultrasound system. To evaluate proper growth, various ratios are used in determining intrauterine growth restriction (IUGR). A common ratio used to estimate proportional growth is femur length to abdominal circumference.

Abdominal Circumference

The AC is used to evaluate fetal growth and fetal age. This measurement is performed by obtaining a transverse image of the fetal abdomen at the level of the stomach and the umbilical vein joining the portal vein, which forms a "J" shape (**FIGURES 5-7** and **5-8**) (AIUM, 2018).

To obtain this level, image the fetus in a longitudinal axis, turn the transducer into a transverse position at the level of the stomach, and then move the transducer superior and inferior until the correct

fetal anatomic landmarks are seen. Note that if the fetal kidneys are visualized, the level is too low in the fetal abdomen. Next, place one caliper on the outside of the anterior skin edge of the abdomen and the other caliper on the outside skin edge of the posterior spine. Open and expand the ellipse to cover the outer portion of the abdomen, including the skin line. The resulting value is calculated by the ultrasound system, and then will provide the estimated gestational age.

Fetal Weight and Growth Predictions

The EFW is obtained by utilizing combinations of fetal anatomic measurements, such as the AC and BPD measurements or the AC and FL measurements. The estimated gestational age and weight are then plotted on a growth chart. Fetal growth charts were created in the 1970s and 1980s, but in most situations are still valid (Kurmananvicius, Burkhardt, Wisser, & Huch, 2004). Most recently, the World Health Organization (2017) reported on their development of an international growth chart that can be used for more diverse populations.

Today, instead of the clinician needing to plot the measurements on a graph, the software in the ultrasound machine often performs the calculations and then displays the results on the report page along with the estimated gestational age and estimated date of delivery.

Formulas that use three measurements, such as HC, AC, and FL, to calculate EFW are available in some software packages that come with the newer ultrasound machines. In some cases, they have proved to be more accurate. Historically, the Hadlock calculations have been generally recognized as most accurate over the full range of fetal weights from 500 to 5000 g (Kurmananvicius et al., 2004). More recently, Cawyer et al. (2018) compared these traditional calculations to the results of new regression-derived formulas that use the average gestational ages calculated for each fetal biometric measurement; they found that the regression formula showed fewer estimates outside the margin of error. The next step in this area is to introduce the regression formula into the ultrasound computer software (Cawyer et al., 2018).

If a fetus is being evaluated for a growth concern, the comparative scans should be performed more than 3 weeks apart (ACOG, 2016b; AIUM, 2018), with the results then being plotted on growth charts (like those shown in the *Sample Estimated Fetal Weight Charts* appendix). A growth scan performed sooner than the recommended 3-week interval can yield erroneous results, which can then snowball, impacting the rest of the pregnancy as well as the outcome.

Depending on the variables present at the time of the scan (such as large for gestational age [LGA], small for gestational age [SGA], preterm premature rupture of membranes [PPROM], or diabetes mellitus), fetal weight predictions may have an error rate as high as $\pm 15\%$ (AIUM 2018). A study by Ben-Haroush et al. (2004) showed that EFW by sonogram had a high correlation with actual birth weight, except in PROM and LGA fetuses. Melamed et al. (2016) found that in SGA fetuses, the current growth charts have significant errors; the same group noted that subgroup-specific models may improve the weight accuracy. Faschingbauer et al. (2016) developed a new formula for SGA that differentiated between symmetric and asymmetric growth patterns that significantly improved the weight estimations. In the PPROM cases, an underestimated EFW occurred; in the LGA cases, an overestimation occurred.

As for pregnancies complicated by diabetes mellitus, Valent et al. (2017) found that although diabetes mellitus affected thoracoabdominal size,

there was no clinically significant alteration in EFW prediction when the ultrasound was performed within 14 days delivery; moreover, the prediction was highly specific for birth weights greater than 4000 g.

Two terms are applied to excessive fetal growth, although they may not be considered universally acceptable: (1) large for gestational age (birth weight greater than or equal to 90th percentile at a specific gestational age) and (2) macrosomia (growth beyond 4000 g or 4500 g regardless of gestational age). However, based on an extensive review of the literature, ACOG has stated ultrasound determination of fetal macrosomia is imprecise with biometry being no better than maternal abdominal palpation (2016c).

Ghi et al. (2016) used quantile regression analysis to develop customizable fetal growth charts based on the parents' height and weight, race, and parity. They were able to define individualized normal ranges of fetal biometric parameters. These researchers found that paternal and maternal height were significant covariates for all measurements, and that maternal weight significantly affected head and abdominal circumference, as well as femur length. Although this study was limited by the racial groups studied, its application can be significant in any country with high immigration rates and variations in parental weight and height.

Gender is an additional consideration for estimating gestational age and weight. Gender-specific growth charts (found in the *Sample Estimated Fetal Weight Charts* appendix) may be used to optimize the prediction of EFW (Schild et al., 2004; Schwarzler et al., 2004). This relationship was further substantiated by Melamed et al. (2013), whose study showed that female fetuses grow considerably more slowly than male fetuses from an early gestation onward. In this study, the female fetus did not appear to be merely a smaller version of the male fetus; instead, the researchers observed a sex-specific growth pattern for each of the individual fetal biometric indices. These findings provide further support for the use of sex-specific sonographic models for fetal weight estimation, as well as the use of sex-specific reference growth charts.

The accuracy of sonographic formulas (Hadlock and Shepard) for estimating weight in singleton gestations was recently studied in twin pregnancies.

All widely used EFW formulas performed equally well in estimating birth weight in twin gestations. However, most women delivered between 33 and 36 weeks' gestation, which limited the studies to gestations of less than 36 weeks (Harper et al., 2013).

The most pertinent point for APs and any sonographer performing ultrasound for estimated fetal age and growth is that when rigorous procedures are used in training sonographers, along with quality assurance oversight, the measurements acquired for singletons can be both accurate and reliable in determining fetal growth (Hediger et al., 2016). As is true with all technology, the accuracy of the results is dependent on the education and training of the person whose hand is on the transducer.

The Fetal Anatomic Survey

A standard sonogram performed after 18 weeks' gestation includes the basic elements of a fetal anatomic screen (**TABLE 5-2**) (ACOG, 2016b; AIUM, 2018). It also includes all of the biometry to determine estimated fetal age and weight, placental location, and amniotic fluid volume; and it may include cervical length. Although anatomic surveys are beyond the scope of ultrasound practice for the majority of APs, deviations from some structural anatomy may be noted during a POC scan, which would indicate the need for appropriate referral. For example, if a complete skull cannot be visualized during a POC scan, that may indicate an anencephalic fetus. The AP would not be responsible for diagnosing the skull defect, but may be responsible for noting there was not a complete skull or that he or she was unable to visualize a complete skull, and that such findings mandate referral and further testing.

▶ Deviations from Normal Fetal Anatomy

Although the elements of the fetal anatomic screen are not a part of a POC or limited sonogram, knowing the normal ultrasound appearance of specific fetal landmarks is imperative to facilitate obtaining the anatomic landmarks for fetal biometry used in estimating fetal age and weight. One method for

TABLE 5-2 Minimal Elements of a Standard Examination of Fetal Anatomy			
Head, face, neck	Cerebellum Choroid plexus Cisterna magna Lateral cerebral ventricles Midline falx Cavum septi pellucidi Upper lip	**Spine**	Cervical, thoracic, lumbar, and sacral spine
Chest	Four-chamber view Left ventricular outflow tract Right ventricular outflow tract	**Extremities**	Presence/absence of legs and arms
Abdomen	Stomach (presence, size, and situs) Kidneys Urinary bladder Umbilical cord insertion site into fetal abdomen Umbilical cord vessel number	**Sex**	Multiple gestations and when medically indicated

Modified from AIUM (2018) and ACOG (2017)

learning normal sonographic anatomy is to compare it with abnormal sonographic anatomic features. This section describes a few significant anatomic abnormalities and presents images to help the practitioner compare normal and abnormal anatomy.

Fetal Head

The fetal cranium normally appears as a hyperechoic oval. Anencephaly is identified by sonography when the fetal cranium cannot be visualized. The most common appearance involves the absence of the cranium from the forehead up, along with the appearance of bulging orbits (**FIGURE 5-9**), which are hypoechoic on sonography.

Lateral Ventricles

At the superior level of the head are the lateral ventricles. The choroid plexus is located within the ventricles and produces cerebral spinal fluid (CSF). The ventricles carry the CSF through the brain. The lateral ventricles are divided into various portions: the frontal, the body, and the occipital. They are located anteriorly, at midportion, and posteriorly, respectively.

It is recommended that the lateral ventricular measurement be taken at the level of the atria to evaluate for hydrocephalus and other anomalies such as Dandy-Walker malformation (**FIGURE 5-10**). This measurement can be routinely obtained after 12 weeks' gestation. The normal measurement should not be greater than 10 mm.

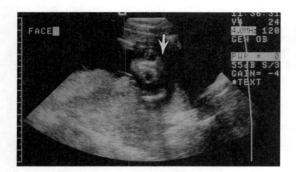

FIGURE 5-9 Anencephaly. Note that the cranium is not over the eyes (at arrows). The eyes appear hypoechoic.

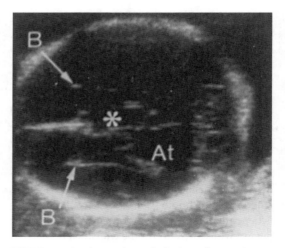

FIGURE 5-10 Axial scan through the lateral ventricles showing typical enlargement of the atria (At) and widely separated bodies (B) with the upward displacement of the third ventricle (*).

Choroid Plexus

The choroid plexus consists of hyperechoic, homogeneous tissue and should be evaluated for simple cysts. Single cysts or multiple cysts creating a mottled appearance to the choroid plexus can be seen before 22 weeks but should resolve after that point in gestation.

Cerebellum

The cerebellum is located in the posterior–inferior portion of the brain. It is imaged by placing the transducer in a coronal position at the frontal bone and angling it posterior to the base of the skull (**FIGURE 5-11** and **FIGURE 5-12**). The transducer may also be angled inferior to the BPD/HC measurement level. Measuring the cerebellum is helpful in determining gestational age.

The cerebellum is responsible for the coordination of muscular movements. The shape of the cerebellum is also important. The normal cerebellum is dumbbell-shaped, similar to that seen in Figure 5-8. If the cerebellum is "banana-shaped," that finding can be indicative of a neural tube defect (the "banana sign"). This abnormality, along with dilated lateral ventricles, is known as a Chiari

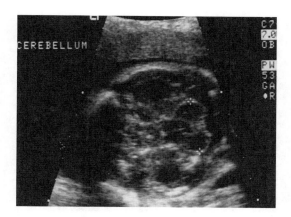

FIGURE 5-11 Cerebellum, between "+" signs.

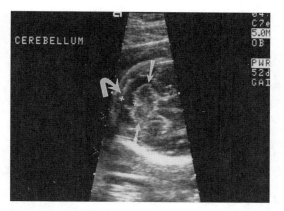

FIGURE 5-12 Cisterna magna (curved arrow) with the measurement between the "+" signs. The cerebellum is between the straight arrows.

malformation (previously named Arnold Chiari) and is associated with spinal defects.

Cerebellar measurements can also be used in cases of suspected symmetric growth restriction to differentiate IUGR from an SGA fetus. The cerebellum is often the last anatomic feature to be compromised in the setting of IUGR.

Cisterna Magna

Posterior to the cerebellum is the cisternal magna, which normally measures 2 to 10 mm (Figure 5-12). This measurement may also be helpful in evaluating

for Dandy-Walker malformation. Also, the cisterna magna will be obliterated in the setting of Chiari malformations and many neural tube defects.

Spine

The spine is divided into five segments: cervical, thoracic, lumbar, sacral, and coccyx. This structure can be evaluated using longitudinal, transverse, and coronal views. The spine is typically ossified after 15 weeks' gestation and, depending on fetal position, can be visualized at this age. To evaluate for spinal closure, a careful scan of each vertebrae, as well as the skin line, is performed in the transverse position. This position permits visualization of the three ossification centers (**FIGURE 5-13**). Any splaying of the ossification centers indicates an abnormality. The longitudinal plane is helpful for imaging and evaluating a complete skin line, as well as the normal spinal curvatures (**FIGURES 5-14**, **5-15**, and **5-16**).

Abnormalities such as cystic hygroma and encephalocele can be identified at the level of the cervical spine. The most common locations for spina bifida and myelomeningocele are the lumbar and sacral spine, although they can occur at any level. Sacrococcygeal teratomas occur at the sacrum and coccyx. Due to these abnormalities, skin closure over the vertebrae is important to image and observe (**FIGURE 5-17**).

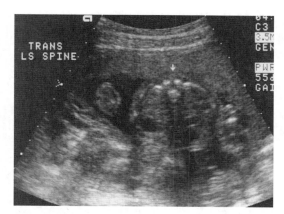

FIGURE 5-13 Transverse view of the spine. The arrow indicates the ossification centers, which in this image are normal.

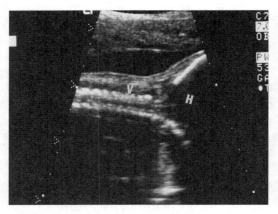

FIGURE 5-14 Longitudinal view of cervical spine. H, head; V, vertebrae.

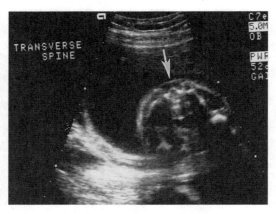

FIGURE 5-17 Transverse view of the lumbar–sacral spine. Note the intact skin closure (arrow).

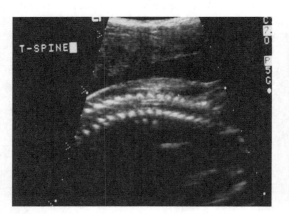

FIGURE 5-15 Thoracic spine in longitudinal view.

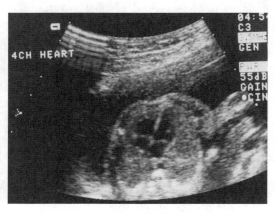

FIGURE 5-18 Axial view of four-chamber fetal heart.

Chest and Heart

The heart is imaged in an axial approach allowing visualization of the four chambers (**FIGURE 5-18**). The heart should make up one-third of the fetal chest. Fetal heart motion is confirmed using M-mode sonography, and this view is then archived to facilitate later comparisons (**FIGURE 5-19**).

Abdomen

The structures in the fetal abdomen that need to be identified during the sonographic evaluation are the stomach, three-vessel umbilical cord, bowel, liver, and gallbladder. One important landmark is the fetal

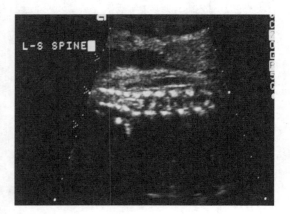

FIGURE 5-16 Lumbar–sacral spine in longitudinal view.

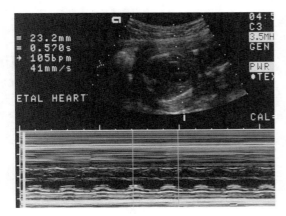

FIGURE 5-19 M-mode tracing of fetal heart verifying cardiac motion.

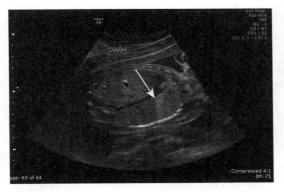

FIGURE 5-20 Longitudinal view of the fetal chest and abdomen. Note the diaphragm (arrow) separating the abdominal contents from the chest contents.

diaphragm (**FIGURE 5-20**), which divides the contents of the abdomen from the chest. The diaphragm is also a useful landmark in the observation of fetal breathing movements during a biophysical profile (see the *Ultrasound Evaluation of Fetal Well-Being* chapter). Since the normal stomach is filled with fluid, sonographically it will appear anechoic (Figure 5-8). It remains this way until term, when the fetus may swallow amniotic fluid containing meconium and/or vernix, which will then appear as hyperechoic debris within the stomach. A left-sided stomach position needs to be confirmed at each sonogram.

The three-vessel umbilical cord is identified in the transverse view. It contains one larger vessel, the umbilical vein, and two smaller vessels, the umbilical arteries (**FIGURE 5-21**). A two-vessel cord would be considered an abnormality and requires further investigation of all other systems.

The umbilical vein enters the abdomen and joins the portal vein in the liver. The umbilical arteries originate at the fetal iliac arteries, extend along each side of the fetal bladder to the anterior abdominal wall, and return to the placenta. The cord insertion site is at the level where the arteries and vein are viewed entering the abdomen (**FIGURE 5-22**). This is a vital image, necessary to assess for abdominal wall defects such as gastroschisis and omphalocele.

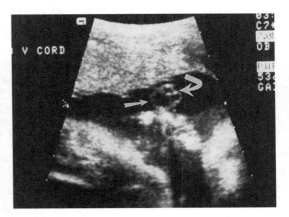

FIGURE 5-21 Transverse view of three-vessel umbilical cord. The large arrow points at the large hypoechoic umbilical vein; the curved arrow indicates the two smaller hypoechoic arteries.

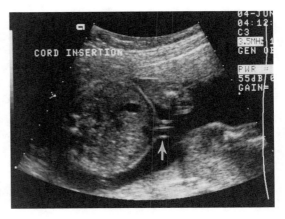

FIGURE 5-22 Cord insertion into the fetal abdomen (arrow).

The fetal gallbladder appears as an ovoid, fluid-filled, tear-drop–shaped structure to the right and inferior to the intrahepatic section of the umbilical vein. It can also be visualized, but may be confused with the umbilical vein due to their proximity. Nonetheless, the gallbladder should be imaged.

Kidneys

Beginning at approximately 16 weeks' gestation, the fetal kidneys may be visualized and evaluated transabdominally. They are located inferior to the level of the stomach. The kidneys are viewed in a transverse approach and are located on either side of the spine (**FIGURE 5-23**). Both the right and left kidneys should be visualized. The kidneys are evaluated for hydronephrosis and cystic or solid masses. A longitudinal or coronal view of the kidneys will assist in differentiating the kidneys from the adrenal glands, which are located cephalad to the kidneys.

Bladder

The fetal bladder is identified as an anechoic structure located between the iliac crests (**FIGURE 5-24**). The bladder will change in volume during the course of the sonogram. This filling and emptying of the bladder will verify that the bladder is free of urethral obstruction.

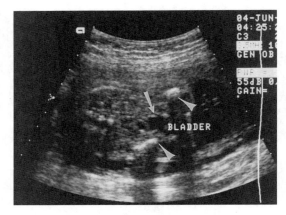

FIGURE 5-24 Fetal bladder (arrow) between the iliac crests (arrowheads).

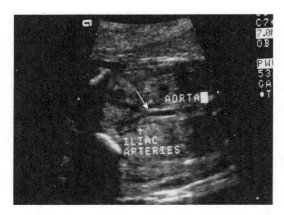

FIGURE 5-25 Fetal aorta (anechoic tubular structure) and iliac arteries branching from it.

Other Views and Measurements

The aorta and iliac arteries may be visualized to assess fetal circulation (**FIGURE 5-25**).

Sex can be difficult to determine in a breech position. Determination of the sex can be done by viewing between both femurs (**FIGURE 5-26**). However, it is possible to misidentify a segment of umbilical cord as a penis (**FIGURE 5-27**).

The nose and lips are very important views in determining facial defects, such as cleft lip and palate. Evaluation of the hands consists of counting digits and identifying normal hand position (**FIGURE 5-28**). The feet can also be evaluated for evidence of clubbing.

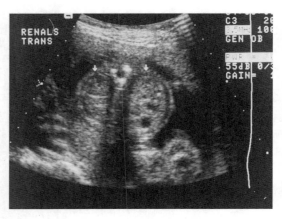

FIGURE 5-23 Transverse view of the fetal kidneys (arrows).

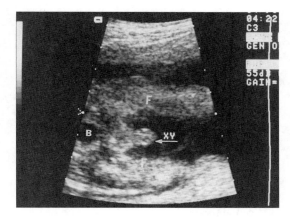

FIGURE 5-26 Male fetus. The penis is identified between the femur bones of each leg. F, femur; bones, xy, penis; B, bladder.

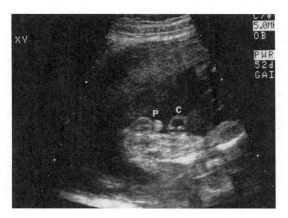

FIGURE 5-27 Differentiation between the umbilical cord (C), which can be between the legs, and the penis (P).

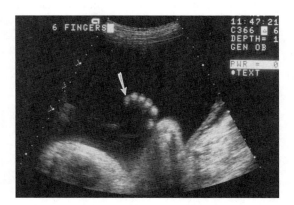

FIGURE 5-28 Fetal hand digits. Arrow indicates polydactyly (six fingers).

Sonographic Assessment of Amniotic Fluid

Amniotic fluid assessment is part of the standard obstetric ultrasound examination. It may be performed subjectively and described with such terms as "increased," "normal," or "decreased." When objective fluid assessments are done during the standard second- and third-trimester sonograms or during a biophysical profile (BPP), the maximum vertical pocket measurement, 2 cm "deepest" pocket, or amniotic fluid index (AFI) may be used (see the *Evaluation of Fetal Well-Being* chapter) (AIUM, 2018). ACOG recommends using objective measurements of amniotic fluid in the third trimester, as well as using the vertical pocket measurement over the AFI when making the diagnosis of oligohydramnios during a BPP (2016b).

The Placenta

Placental localization is part of the standard second- and third-trimester obstetric sonograms. The placental appearance and location in relationship to the cervical os should be documented (AIUM, 2018). The sonographic appearance of placental tissue begins as echogenic focal thickening of the wall of the gestational sac early in pregnancy, then proceeds to a more homogenous appearance toward the end of the first trimester that continues throughout the duration of the pregnancy. Hyperechoic lines of calcification may be seen outlining the cotyledons as the placenta matures. The placental location, appearance, and proximity to the cervical os should be observed and documented (ACOG, 2016b).

POC or limited ultrasound of the placenta is indicated when a woman presents in the second or third trimester with a chief complaint of vaginal bleeding. Differential diagnosis of bleeding in pregnancy includes such etiologies as placental abruption and placenta previa, but other causes may include cervical erosion, preterm labor, term labor, and lacerations, to name a few. Diagnosis of placental-related bleeding issues has significantly improved since the introduction of ultrasound into obstetric care (AIUM, 2018; Williams, Laifer-Narin, & Ragavendra, 2003). Because spotting or bleeding in pregnancy is a frequent cause of urgent care visits, this next section focuses on placental abruption, placenta previa, and other placental deviations that carry the risk for adverse maternal and fetal conditions.

Placenta Previa

Placenta previa refers to placental tissue that covers or partially covers the internal cervical os. The patient classically presents with painless vaginal bleeding. The incidence of placenta previa is 1 in 200 to 250 births. Of those cases, approximately 20% are complete previas and 80% are marginal or partial previas. In recent years, there has been an increased incidence of placenta implantation defects directly related to the increased incidence of cesarean births, with the placenta implanting into the cesarean section scar, known as placenta accreta (ACOG, 2017). Potential complications from placenta previa include premature delivery and hemorrhage.

To avoid errors in sonographic interpretation, both the lower edge of the placenta and the internal cervical os must be visualized. In a study by Rosati and Guariglia (2000), transvaginal sonography (TVS) was used as the primary method for evaluating placental location in 10- to 16-week gestations. Although there was a high false-positive rate (placenta previa diagnosed by the early scan but not present later in pregnancy), the transvaginal (TV) approach can be effective in high-risk patients. TVS permits specific measurements from the lower margin of the placenta to the internal os. However, care must be taken not to apply the pressure of the transducer to the cervix or lower uterine segment, because doing so could potentially cause bleeding or an error in measurement. The transperineal approach may be a safer option.

When a previa is diagnosed early in pregnancy, follow-up scans are imperative (ACOG, 2016b; Rosati & Guariglia, 2000). Care must be taken not to misinterpret an echogenic subchorionic hematoma overlying the cervix for placental tissue. Sonographically, placenta previa appears as placental tissue covering all or part of the internal cervical os. This tissue may be normal echogenic placental tissue or

hypoechoic venous lakes or vessels of the placenta. There may be displacement of the presenting fetal part from the internal os. Placenta previa can be excluded if one of the following can be demonstrated:

- Direct sonographic visualization of both the lower edge of the placenta and the internal cervical os, with the lower edge of the placenta seen separate from the cervix
- Amniotic fluid between the presenting part and the cervix without interposed placental tissue, or the presenting part immediately overlying the cervix without space for intervening placental tissue

Ultrasound diagnosis of placenta previa is divided into the following categories based on the placental proximity to the cervical os: (1) a complete previa covers the entire internal os, (2) a partial previa covers only a section of the internal os of the cervix, and (3) a low-lying (marginal) placenta is defined as the placental margin being located 2 cm or less from the internal os of the cervix (Johnson & Kutz, 2018). This is important to recognize because a low-lying placenta frequently requires a cesarean birth due to bleeding at the time of delivery, therefore it must be reported to the provider.

Distinguishing an asymmetric complete placenta previa from a partial placenta previa or a very low-lying placenta may be difficult. If a low-lying placenta or placenta previa is suspected early in gestation, verification in the third trimester by repeat ultrasonography is indicated. In women who have had a prior cesarean section, if an anterior placenta previa or low-lying placenta is visualized, the possibility of an abnormal placental implantation such as placenta accreta is increased and, therefore, warrants heightened concern (ACOG, 2016; ACOG, 2017).

Total placental previa occurs when the placenta completely covers the cervical os. The placenta may be predominately on the anterior, posterior, or lateral uterine wall extending over the cervix, but often is not symmetrically located over the cervical os (**FIGURE 5-29**). When the placenta is concentrically implanted about the cervical os, the term *central placenta previa* is frequently used.

TVS has also shown to be very effective in the diagnosis of placenta previa. This type of sonography

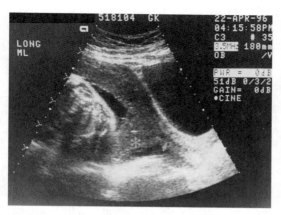

FIGURE 5-29 Complete placenta previa. Internal cervical os (small arrow); placenta (*).

permits specific measurements to be made from the lower margin of the placenta to the internal os. Care must be taken to ensure that the maternal bladder is empty and that the sonographer not apply transducer pressure to the cervix or lower uterine segment, because it could potentially cause bleeding or cause error in measurement.

A partial or marginal placenta previa that is seen during the second trimester should be sonographically reevaluated in the third trimester of pregnancy. Many times, the uterus has grown in such a manner that the placenta is no longer as close to or covering the internal cervical os. This movement of the placenta is referred to as *placental migration*. The apparent movement or motion appears to be a result of differential growth rates between the lower uterine segment and the placenta, with relatively rapid growth of the myometrium just above the level of the cervix.

Technical factors that can mimic placenta previa include focal uterine contractions and an overly distended bladder. A focal uterine contraction can be suspected if the myometrial wall is focally thickened (more than 1.5 cm). The placenta is usually more echogenic than the contracted uterine wall. Rescanning after 30 to 60 minutes generally allows sufficient time for the contraction to dissipate and to restore the normal anatomic relationships.

During a transabdominal scan, an overly distended bladder may press against the lower uterine segment, bringing the anterior wall against the posterior wall and causing an artificially elongated cervix. If the cervix measures greater than 3 to 4 cm, then the bladder is probably overdistended. If this occurs, the woman can partially void, with the sonogram then being repeated. If the placental location in relationship to the cervix still cannot be determined, have the patient void completely and repeat the sonogram. If the cervical os cannot be adequately identified using the transabdominal ultrasound technique, TV or transperineal techniques may be used.

An alternative method of evaluating the internal cervical os is the transperineal or translabial approach. It requires no specialized equipment or vaginal penetration. The bladder is emptied, and the woman is placed in the lithotomy position. A sector (abdominal) transducer that is covered with an appropriate cover is placed in the sagittal orientation directly over or between the labia minora. The transducer is angled medially and laterally to image the entire internal surface of the cervix. The orientation of the image will be the same as with the TV transducer: The vagina is at the apex of the image (top of the screen), and the cervix is in a horizontal plane.

Vasa Previa. Vasa previa occurs when unprotected fetal blood vessels run through the amniotic membranes and traverse the cervical os. A vasa previa may present as one of two types: (1) a velamentous insertion, which is when there are unprotected fetal blood vessels traversing the cervical os that are inserted into the membrane between the umbilical cord and the placenta, or (2) when there is a succenturiate lobe, multilobe, or bilobe with fetal blood vessels connecting the two placental lobes which are near or over the (Society for Maternal-Fetal Medicine [SMFM], 2015).

The rate of occurrence has been reported as 1 in 2500 (0.002%) births (SMFM, 2015), but there are reports as high as 1 out of approximately 1600 (0.001%) births to as low as 1 out of 3000 (0.003%) births. Albeit extraordinarily rare, it carries a 56% perinatal death rate when it has not been antenatally identified (Kulkarni et al., 2018). These unsupported vessels are prone to tearing when the membranes rupture, resulting in fetal exsanguination and death in at least 75% of the cases. There also may be compression of vessels by a presenting part, which compromises feto-placental circulation. The highly significant association between a second-trimester placenta previa and vasa previa at birth further supports the need for follow-up sonographic evaluation of early scans that demonstrate a placenta previa (Francois, Mayer, Harris, & Perlow, 2003; SMFM, 2015).

This condition is the result of the velamentous insertion of the umbilical cord in the lower uterine segment so that the unsupported cord vessels traverse through membranes and across the internal cervical os (**FIGURE 5-30**).

The location of the cord insertion into the fetal abdomen is an integral part of all obstetric sonographic studies (ACOG, 2018; AIUM, 2018) and can assist with determining the presence or absence of a vasa previa. Color Doppler ultrasound is extremely helpful in making the diagnosis of both vasa previa and velamentous insertion of the cord because of its ability to accurately determine the cord insertion site. If an abnormal cord insertion or any placental abnormality is noted, such as an extra lobe, a TV scan should be performed to further evaluate for any abnormality. Interestingly, Kulkarni et al. (2018) recently reported that *routine* ultrasound screening for vasa previa following AIUM scanning criteria can prevent such perinatal mortality.

Morbidly Adherent Placenta

Morbidly adherent placenta (MAP), also known as a placenta accreta, is an abnormal attachment of the placenta in which the chorionic villi have grown directly into the myometrium and perhaps further. Accretas are classified into three categories depending on the extension of their growth. If the villi have grown only into the myometrium, the condition is called *placenta accreta vera*. This type of accreta is attributed to complete or partial absence of the decidua basalis and imperfect development of the fibrin layer. If the villi have penetrated deeper into the myometrium, the condition is called *placenta increta*. If the uterine serosa has been penetrated, the villi may pass through the uterus and often attach into the bladder or rectum (Moore & Gonzalez, 2008). This condition is referred to as *placenta percreta* (**FIGURES 5-31** and **5-32**). The newer term,

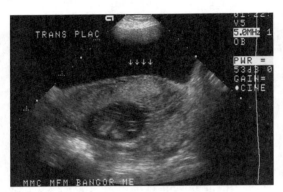

FIGURE 5-31 Transverse transabdominal image of placenta accreta (arrows pointing to invasion).

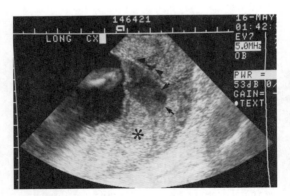

FIGURE 5-30 Variation of vasa previa. Transvaginal sonography demonstrates a large area of vascularity by the internal cervical os. Vasa previa (arrows); internal cervical os (arrows); internal cervical os (arrowheads); placenta (*).

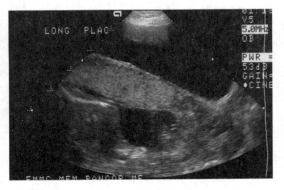

FIGURE 5-32 Sagittal view of the placenta accreta shown in Figure 5-31.

morbidly adherent placenta, encompasses all of these distinctions, in recognition of the fact that an abnormally attached placenta of any depth increases maternal morbidity and mortality (ACOG, 2017).

The most common predisposing factor for developing placenta accreta or MAP is the presence of a uterine scar from previous cesarean birth. Placenta accreta can cause antepartum bleeding, but in the majority of cases the bleeding is a consequence of coexisting placenta previa. The greatest risk associated with placenta accreta occurs during the third stage of labor, when the placenta may fail to separate and deliver, resulting in persistent postpartum bleeding and maternal hemorrhage. Severe hemorrhage, uterine perforation, and infection resulting from attempts at manual removal contribute to maternal morbidity and mortality. If manual extraction is unsuccessful, a surgical intervention may be necessary to control bleeding.

At times, placenta accreta may be visualized by ultrasound by analyzing the retroplacental complex. A normal placental attachment site is characterized by a hypoechoic boundary between the placenta and the bladder. In accreta, this band is either absent or less than 2 mm thick. Additionally, there is a loss of the normal decidual interface between the placenta and the myometrium with an increasing number of placental lakes (lacunae), appearing as "Swiss cheese" or "moth eaten." If the placenta is located posteriorly, a TV ultrasound with Doppler or magnetic resonance imaging (MRI) should be utilized (ACOG, 2017; Doshe & Hoffman, 2016; Moore & Gonzalez, 2008).

Other sonographic markers of MAP include the following:

- Absence or severe thinning of the hypoechoic myometrium between the placenta and uterine serosa–bladder wall complex
- Thinning, irregularity, or disruption of the linear hypoechoic uterine serosa–bladder wall complex
- Extension of tissue of placental echogenicity beyond the uterine serosa

Placental Abruption

Placenta abruption is also referred to as *placenta abruption*, *abruptio placentae*, *ablatio placentae*, and *premature separation* or *abnormally implanted placenta*. Sonographic examination is not as sensitive for the detection of an abruption as it is for a placenta previa. Because of the stages of evolution of a hematoma (fresh bleeding, clotting, hematoma formation, etc.), if the ultrasound is performed when the hematoma is isoechoic as is the placenta, it may be missed. Therefore, what might appear to be normal does not completely exclude a placental abruption. However, when a positive finding is noted, such as visualization of a hematoma, then the likelihood of an abruption increases (Shinde, Vaswani, Patange, Laddad, & Bhosale, 2018).

The sonographic appearance of an abruption depends on its age. An acute hematoma may range from hyperechoic to isoechoic relative to the placenta. A resolving hematoma generally becomes hypoechoic or will have mixed echoes within a week of the onset of symptoms. This depends on the degree of organization. Within 2 weeks, the resolving hematoma will be anechoic (**FIGURES 5-33** and **5-34**). Color Doppler may be useful to determine a suspected abruption. The color Doppler box is positioned over the anatomic area of interest. The color filter is then adjusted to the most sensitive low-flow setting, and the Doppler velocity scale to the low- or slow-flow setting. The presence of color flow in the suspected area will rule out abruption.

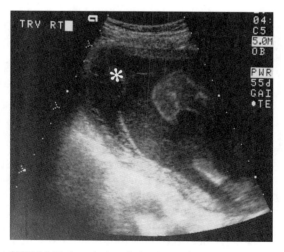

FIGURE 5-33 Isoechoic subchorionic abruption (*).

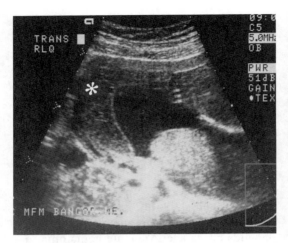

FIGURE 5-34 The same patient as in Figure 5-33, 18 days later. Note the mixed echogenicity of the abruption (*).

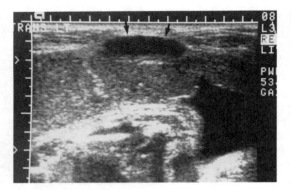

FIGURE 5-35 Retroplacental abruption demonstrating bleeding with the separation of the placenta from the uterine wall (arrows).

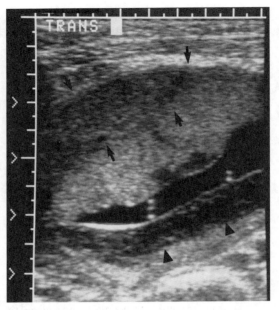

FIGURE 5-36 Retroplacental abruption (arrows) demonstrating a biconcave appearance. Subchorionic bleeding is noted (arrowheads).

The color Doppler settings should be readjusted and the area of interest reimaged if no flow is demonstrated. Color amplitude power mapping, when available, is also helpful in visualizing flow. The probability of an abruption is greatly increased if flow is not demonstrated using these techniques.

Abruption may be categorized as retroplacental, subchorionic and marginal, or preplacental. Retroplacental abruption occurs when the placenta separates from the myometrial wall (**FIGURE 5-35**). Evidence suggests that retroplacental abruption usually results from the rupture of the decidual spiral arteries, with hemorrhage into the decidua

basalis producing "high-pressure" bleeds. Most small retroplacental hematomas are asymptomatic, whereas large hematomas may have devastating consequences. Retroplacental hematomas are often linear or biconcave with well-defined margins (**FIGURE 5-36**). Large hematomas may deform the overlying placenta and produce bulging of the chorionic plate.

Acute retroplacental hematomas may be difficult to recognize because they dissect into the placenta and/or myometrium and are isoechoic to the adjacent placenta. In these cases, sonography may demonstrate a thickened, heterogenous-appearing placenta that may measure up to 9 cm thick, compared to a normal thickness of 4 to 5 cm.

With the finding of a thickened, heterogenous-appearing placenta, the differential diagnosis includes (1) normal retroplacental myometrium with prominent basal veins, (2) retroplacental myoma, (3) myometrial contraction, and (4) placental maturation along the basal plate. When an abruption is diagnosed by ultrasound, follow-up sonograms are recommended to ensure that the placental abruption decreases in size and that fetal growth is appropriate for gestational age. Other fetal testing may be indicated.

A marginal placental abruption is seen at the periphery of the placenta and can result from tears of marginal veins, which produce "low-pressure" bleeds. This most likely occurs because the placental membrane separates more easily from the myometrium than does the more firmly attached placenta. The placental edge is elevated slightly, but marginal abruption is associated with little placental detachment and clinical symptoms are mild. The hematoma may extend away from the placenta to the subchorionic area.

In some situations, a subchorionic hematoma may be seen in a site remote from the placenta and is presumed to have originated from bleeding at the placental margin (**FIGURE 5-37**). Nearly all subchorionic hematomas arise from marginal abruptions,

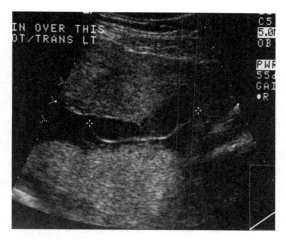

FIGURE 5-38 Preplacental bleeding with blood between the placenta and chorion anechoic area noted between **.

but in only half of the cases is placental detachment demonstrated by ultrasound. As the hematoma resolves, the detached placental membrane may be the only evidence of prior subchorionic hematoma.

The sonographic differential diagnosis with this type of abruption includes succenturiate lobe, chorioangioma, placenta previa, and coexisting molar pregnancy.

Preplacental abruption occurs when blood collects between the placenta and the chorion, or between the amnion and the chorion, although the distinction between the two usually cannot be made by ultrasound (**FIGURE 5-38**). Large preplacental hematomas may produce clinical symptoms similar to placental abruption, but placental detachment does not occur from preplacental hematomas.

Differentiating Placental Tissue from Other Structures

Unusual shapes or configurations of the placenta will impact the sonographic appearance of the structure and may impact birth outcome. A succenturiate or bilobed placenta (**FIGURE 5-39**) is an accessory lobe connected by either blood vessels within a membrane or by chorionic tissue to the main placental mass. Risks associated with this condition include retained placental tissue and fetal

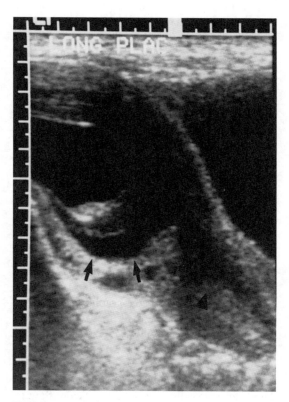

FIGURE 5-37 Subchorionic hematoma with blood (arrows) at the internal os (arrowhead).

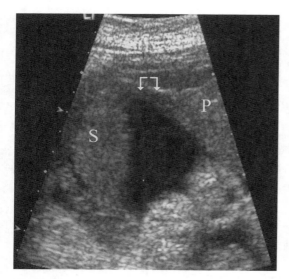

FIGURE 5-39 Succenturiate lobe. The succenturiate lobe (S) is connected to the placenta (P) by the bridge of tissue and vessels.

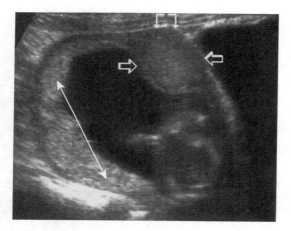

FIGURE 5-40 Differentiation between a fibroid (between arrowheads) and placental tissue along the right lateral uterine wall; the double arrow indicates placental tissue. Note the differences in the types of echoes, with the fibroid appearing more isoechoic.

hemorrhage. A circumvallate placenta is defined as placental implantation that extends beyond the limits of the chorionic plate. Other deviations from normal include amniotic bands, as well as abnormal placental size as seen in fetal hydrops.

Placental tissue must also be differentiated from leiomyomas (fibroids) (**FIGURE 5-40**) and uterine

contraction. Fibroids often distort the wall of the uterus and alter the contour. On the other hand, uterine contractions can be determined either by palpation of the maternal abdomen or by continued sonographic observation until the contraction ends and the "mass" disappears.

Placental Calcifications

As the placenta matures, some degree of calcification occurs, which appears sonographically as hyperechoic "patches." This calcification formed the basis of the placental grading that was once evaluated as the sixth parameter in the biophysical profile (Vintzileos, Campbell, Ingardia, & Nochimson, 1983) (see the *Sonographic Evaluation of Fetal Well-Being* chapter).

Placental Lakes

On examination of the placenta, hypoechoic areas within the placental tissue—known as venous or placental lakes—may be seen. Placental lakes are more likely to be found with a thick placenta (more than 3 cm at 20 weeks' gestation) and do not appear to be associated with uteroplacental complications or adverse pregnancy outcomes (Smith & Smith, 2003; Thompson et al., 2002) in most cases. However, as mentioned previously, increasing numbers of placental lakes may also be an indication of a placental accreta and should be investigated further (Doshe & Hoffman, 2016).

Postpartum Retained Placenta

When clinical suspicions point to possible retained placental products during the postpartum period, a sonogram may be ordered prior to surgical interventions. The sonographic findings are often nonspecific because blood clots and retained products show considerable overlap in their sonographic appearances. The most common finding of retained placental tissue is an endometrial mass (**FIGURE 5-41**) (Durfee, Frates, Luong, & Benson, 2005; Kamaya et al., 2009). The use of color Doppler, however, can further clarify a clot versus retained products. A clot within the endometrium typically does not display color flow. In contrast, retained products often have a "stalk-like" or diffuse flow within the mass or endometrium.

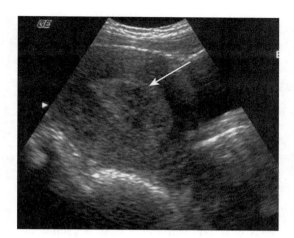

FIGURE 5-41 Retained placental tissue.

Maternal Cervical Length Measurement

Measuring cervical length is performed as part of a standard obstetric sonogram when appropriate (ACOG, 2017; AIUM, 2018), but has also become a relatively common POC or limited sonogram performed in response to a complaint of uterine activity or cramping. Until recently, the research pertaining to the association between cervical length and preterm birth had focused on the high-risk population, particularly women with a history of preterm birth. The benefit of the routine cervical length measurement was clearly established as a predictor for preterm birth in women with a history of prior preterm birth. Crane and Hutchens (2008) showed that cervical length measurement done with TV ultrasound in asymptomatic high-risk women predicted spontaneous preterm birth at less than 35 weeks' gestation.

However, because approximately 50% of preterm births occur in nulliparous women, the need for a screening exam in this group appears to be as important as screening the high-risk group. A study by Cahill et al. (2010) sought to determine a strategy that would be cost-effective for the treatment of preterm birth when a short cervix was diagnosed by ultrasound. The study focused on using ultrasound cervical length measurements as a screening in all pregnant women, rather than scanning only those determined to be at risk based on history. The researchers' conclusion was that universal screening

for cervical length, followed by treatment with progesterone gel of those determined to have a short cervical length, was cost-effective. This approach also resulted in a statistically significant reduction of preterm birth at less than 34 weeks' gestation.

The Cahill et al. study was followed by a study by Hassan et al. (2011) specifically testing the efficacy of progesterone gel in reducing the rate of preterm birth in those women with an ultrasound-diagnosed short cervix between 19 and 23 weeks' gestation. This prospective, randomized, double-blinded study included 44 medical centers in 10 countries. A short cervix was defined as being between 10 and 20 mm in asymptomatic women. The results showed a substantial reduction in the rate of preterm delivery at less than 33 weeks' gestation and a significant decrease in the rate of respiratory distress syndrome (RDS). Based on these studies, many healthcare providers now believe that there is convincing evidence supporting routine cervical length measurements in all pregnant women in the second trimester of pregnancy (Campbell, 2011). Carrying this research one step further, Grobman et al. (2016) attempted to evaluate whether the combination of demographic and sonographic factors associated with nulliparous preterm birth with a cervical length less than 30 mm would accurately predict preterm birth; unfortunately, they found that an accurate prediction model could not be developed based on these factors. Further study is needed before a predictive model can be recommended.

TV cervical ultrasound has been shown to be a reliable and reproducible method for assessing cervical length in the second trimester of pregnancy (ACOG, 2012) and is considered the gold standard (AIUM, 2018; Cervical Length Education and Review [CLEAR], 2018). Transabdominal (TA) cervical length measurements performed with an empty bladder have shown a close correlation with TV ultrasound in some studies and may be the first step in cervical assessment (Chory et al., 2016; Saul, Kurtzman, Hagemann, Ghamsary, & Wing, 2008). In fact, women who have "long" measurements obtained by TA scan may not need follow-up TV scans (Chory et al., 2016). ACOG (2012) also recommends the use of cervical length measurement for determining which patients do *not* need tocolysis: Cervical length ultrasound has a good negative predictive value in showing that those with a normal cervical length will not need tocolysis.

Ultrasound measurement of the cervix is a screening test that will not detect all women at risk for preterm labor. Conversely, many women deemed to be at risk will not deliver preterm even without treatment. Nevertheless, cervical measurement can be helpful in determining when to transfer a patient to a tertiary facility or when to initiate therapies such as progesterone, steroids, tocolysis, or cervical cerclage. Importantly, it can help avoid costly and potentially risky treatments for women who are not likely to benefit from those therapies (e.g., prolonged hospitalization or prolonged home bed rest). The majority of women with symptoms suspicious for preterm labor will not proceed to immediate delivery. Measuring cervical length has been shown to decrease the number of days of hospitalization and decrease the use of medication without increasing the number of preterm births (Ness, Visintine, Ricci, & Berghella, 2007; Sanin-Blair et al., 2004).

In summary, multiple studies have shown that a short cervix measured by ultrasound is a powerful predictor for preterm birth. As recommended by ACOG (2008, 2016a), treatment with injectable progesterone has proved successful in reducing the preterm birth rate in high-risk pregnancies. Therefore, ultrasound measurement of cervical length may be useful in the following clinical situations:

- Evaluate the risk of preterm labor in symptomatic and asymptomatic women.
- Confirm or refute the suspicion of an incompetent cervix.
- Determine whether a woman with symptoms of labor is likely to deliver in the near future, especially if she is preterm.
- Predict the likelihood of a successful induction of labor (Crane & Hutchens, 2008).
- Evaluate the chance of a pregnancy continuing post term.
- Evaluate the risk of cesarean birth (Smith et al., 2008).
- Determine the timing of a maternal transport for women who need to deliver at a distance from their home due to complications of pregnancy or need for immediate neonatal care that is not available locally.

Measuring Cervical Length

Cervical length measurements must be performed following standardized training using proper technique if they are to be predictive (Chory et al., 2016; CLEAR, 2018; Taylor, 2011). Errors in scanning technique that can distort the appearance of the cervix or alter cervical measurements include putting too much pressure against the cervix with the vaginal probe or the use of fundal pressure. An overly distended maternal bladder can also exert enough pressure to artificially elongate the cervix (CLEAR, 2018).

The distal portion of the uterus, the uterine cervix, consists primarily of cartilaginous connective tissue that serves to close the passageway from the uterus to the vagina. It softens with pregnancy, and prior to labor it begins to efface or thin. This process starts from the *inner* os of the cervix, the uterine end of the canal, and progresses toward the external os at the vaginal end (Gramellini et al., 2002; Rust, Atlas, Kimmel, Roberts, & Hess, 2005) (**FIGURES 5-42**, **5-43**, and **5-44**). This internal effacement can be seen by ultrasound, but it cannot be felt by an examining finger (Berghella et al., 1997; Debbs & Chen, 2009) (**FIGURES 5-45** and **5-46**). The uneffaced, closed portion of the cervix can be measured by ultrasound.

Expertise in evaluating the anatomy of the lower uterine segment and cervix can be of value when assessing placental position relative to the cervix. Cervical length can be reliably measured once the lower uterine segment and the cervix can be differentiated. This occurs at approximately

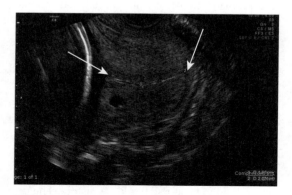

FIGURE 5-42 Cervical length, between arrows.

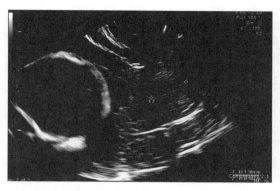

FIGURE 5-43 Cervical length noted between **. Because the cervix is curved, two lengths are determined and then added together.

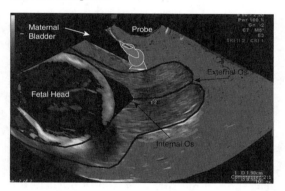

FIGURE 5-44 The same image as in Figure 5-43, but with the lower uterine segment, cervix, and cervical canal outlined for clarity.

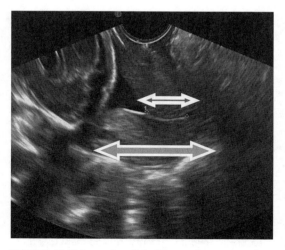

FIGURE 5-45 This cervix will feel longer (large arrows) to palpation than its functional length (small arrows).

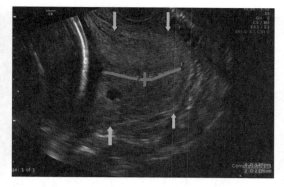

FIGURE 5-46 This cervix will feel shorter (between the arrows) than its functional length (measured in gray).

14 weeks' gestation. Prior to this point in gestation, measuring cervical length is generally not recommended (Berghella, Talucci, & Desai, 2003).

Cervical sonogram is done with a high-frequency vaginal transducer (3 to 9 MHz). Measurement using the abdominal approach has generally not been found to be sufficiently accurate (Berghella & Khalifeh, 2016; CLEAR, 2018), except when the cervix is long, as noted earlier. Although transperineal or translabial methods can be successful, these techniques are more difficult to master and may not always be successful even for the experienced sonographer (Cicero et al., 2001).

The pregnant woman should be reassured that a vaginal ultrasound is no more uncomfortable than a digital examination of the cervix (Taylor, 2011). The woman should have an empty bladder, both for comfort and to prevent elongating the lower uterine segment and causing the cervix to appear longer. The woman can be placed in a supine position with her knees flexed, just as she would for a digital examination of the cervix. It may be helpful to elevate her buttocks with a folded blanket or have her put her fists under her buttocks. Alternatively, she can be placed in lithotomy position with her feet in stirrups, as if for a speculum examination. The transducer should be covered with a probe cover or the finger of an exam glove. A generous amount of gel is applied on the inside and the outside of the probe cover, being careful to avoid air bubbles that will prevent the transmission of the sound waves and obscure the image.

The examiner places his or her thumb on the directional guide on the probe (a notch or groove). The transducer should remain in the 12 o'clock position, which will result in a sagittal section, or a slice parallel to the maternal long axis. The probe should be inserted gently and slowly while watching for the appropriate landmarks as they appear on the monitor. The corner of the maternal bladder and amniotic fluid should be visible. The internal os, the cervical canal, and the anterior and posterior lip of the cervix at the external os should be identifiable (AIUM, 2018). The left side of the screen will be cephalad. The right side will be caudal, extending into the vagina. The internal cervical os will be on the left and the external os on the right. With minimal gentle rocking, tilting, or rotation of the transducer, it should be possible to elongate the entire cervical canal (**FIGURE 5-47**).

An adequate view of the cervix is considered one that is visible on approximately 75% of the image, with the bladder being visibly empty, the anterior and posterior cervical thickness being equal with similar echogenicity, and limited concavity caused by the TV transducer (CLEAR, 2018). If the probe pushes directly on the cervix, it can cause it to elongate, exaggerating its length (Yost, Bloom, Twickler, & Leveno, 1999). Calipers are placed where the walls of the anterior and posterior cervix touch at the internal and external os, not extending to the outermost edge of the cervical tissue. A measurement is then taken from the external os to the internal os of the cervix. The cervical canal is frequently curved, especially when the cervix is long. In such a case, it may be necessary to measure it in two or more separate pieces, with the measurements then being added together (**FIGURE 5-48**). Tracing the canal has been found to be less accurate than summing two straight measurements. If the cervix is short, it will often be straight (CLEAR, 2018). It is also recommended to apply mild suprapubic or fundal pressure for approximately 15 seconds, as this will give another opportunity to view funneling if it has begun (CLEAR, 2018). The length of the cervix may be noted to change during the examination if a uterine contraction occurs. This occasionally may be a dramatic change.

At least three measurements should be taken, and the shortest of the three measurements used so as to err on the side of caution. In other words, the shortest measurement should be reported, because the shorter the cervix, the greater the risk of preterm birth and all the sequelae associated with that event. The shortest measurement is most predictive of preterm birth (Rust et al., 2005). Average cervical length prior to 22 weeks is 40 mm. From 22 to 32 weeks, the average length is 35 mm, and the cervix

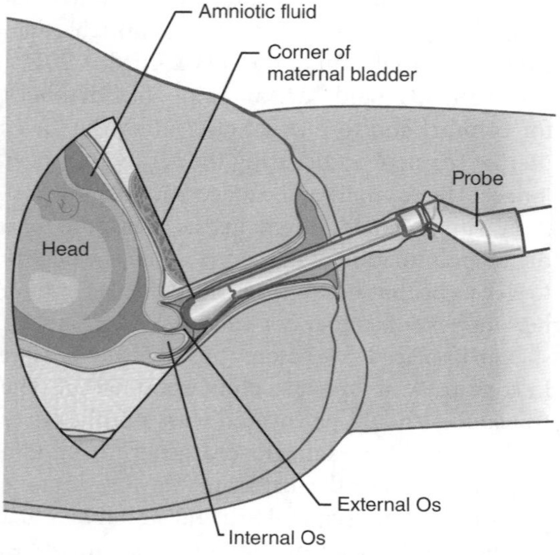

FIGURE 5-47 Proper transvaginal probe placement.

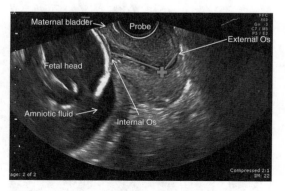

FIGURE 5-48 Curved cervix. In this case, it is better to measure in straight segments and add them together than it is to draw one straight line. A straight line will incorrectly show a shorter length.

will continue to shorten until term. Between 22 and 30 weeks, the 10th percentile for cervical length is 25 mm. A length less than 25 mm was shown to be statistically significant in association with preterm delivery, with the risk increasing as cervical length decreases (ACOG, 2016a; Goldenberg et al., 2003; Mercer et al., 1996). Treatment with progesterone has been shown to be most effective when the cervical length is between 10 and 20 mm (ACOG, 2012; Berghella, 2009).

Because the cervix effaces from the internal os to the external os, it precedes dilation and cannot be palpated by an examining finger. This process creates a characteristic funnel shape or "beaking" appearance that has been described as progressing from a "T" shape, where the amniotic fluid meets the cervical canal, to a "Y" shape, to a "V," and finally to a "U" when membranes are bulging into the cervical canal (although the membranes may not yet be palpable in the vagina) (**FIGURES 5-49, 5-50, 5-51,** and **5-52**). Although funneling is associated with a short cervix and preterm labor, the critical factor in predicting preterm birth is the closed length of the cervix, not the amount of funneling (Berghella et al., 1997; CLEAR, 2018).

When measuring cervical length by ultrasound, follow these guidelines:

- Do not perform the measurement before 14 to 15 weeks' gestation.
- Measure vaginally and not abdominally, when possible.
- Use sufficient gel inside the probe cover to prevent the formation of air pockets, as they will interfere with visualization.
- Do not perform TV measurements with a full maternal bladder.
- Do not apply pressure to the cervix.
- The anterior width of the cervix should equal the posterior width.
- Both the internal os and the external os should be viewed.
- The entire length of the cervical canal should be viewed.
- Do not rush. Allow time for a contraction to occur or subside.

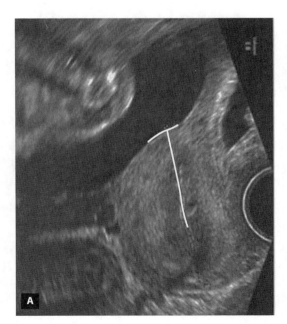
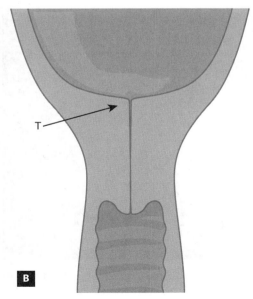

FIGURE 5-49 A. Image of a long and closed cervix, with the internal cervical os closed at the level of the amniotic fluid (the top of the "T" running along this straight edge and the tail of the "T" running through the long cervix). **B.** A schematic diagram illustrating this normal finding.

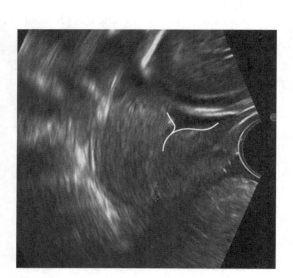

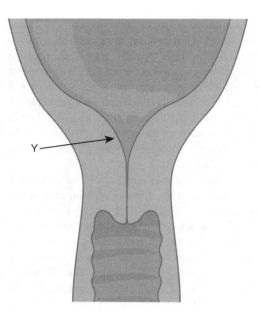

FIGURE 5-50 The internal os is slightly open, changing the "T" more to a "Y."

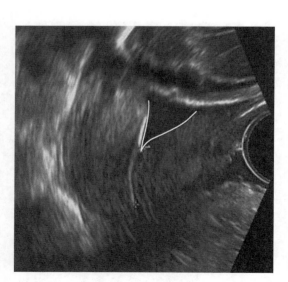

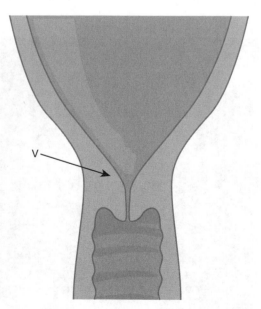

FIGURE 5-51 As the cervix further effaces, the internal os opens and changes from a "Y" shape to a "V" shape. The image shows the anechoic amniotic fluid dipping into the internal os.

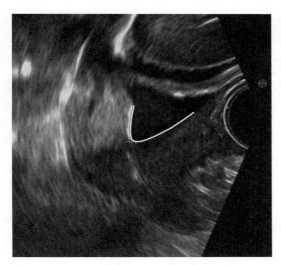 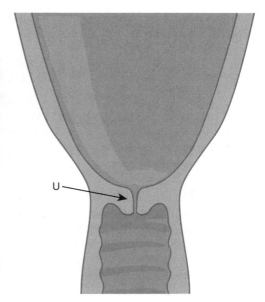

FIGURE 5-52 As the internal os continues to shorten, the amniotic fluid fills the space and forms a "U" appearance, as shown in both the image and the diagram. The arrow is pointing at the uterus.

- Observe the image on the monitor in real time as the probe is inserted.
- The risk assessment is based on the closed cervical length, not the amount of funneling.

In summary, multiple studies have shown that a short cervix measured by ultrasound is a powerful predictor for preterm birth. In high-risk pregnancies, ACOG (2008, 2016a) recommends treatment with injectable progesterone to reduce the preterm birth rate. Additionally, ultrasound measurement of cervical length can be of value in several clinical situations. It is better at predicting who will *not* deliver preterm than who will. POC bedside ultrasound can be a valuable tool for a rapid, painless assessment of the cervix. With experience, education, and training, the total exam time can be approximately 3 to 5 minutes (CLEAR, 2018).

▶ Summary

POC sonography has multiple applications and indications during the second and third trimesters of pregnancy, ranging from determining gestational age and weight to determining placental location and cervical length. Regardless of the indication for POC sonography, there is no doubt that bedside ultrasound has the tremendous potential for saving time and money, as well as promoting quality of care and patient outcome.

Study Questions

1. What is the major difference between a point-of-care (POC) and standard second trimester ultrasound exam?
   a. Placental location
   b. Fetal biometric measurements
   c. Specific fetal anatomic survey

2. What is the appropriate follow-up if a second-trimester ultrasound indicates gestational dating different from the first-trimester dating ultrasound?
   a. Change the estimated due date based on the second-trimester exam.
   b. Repeat the ultrasound in 2 weeks to see if there is still a discrepancy.
   c. Obtain a consultation regarding the plan of management for the dating discrepancy.

3. Which view of the fetal head should be obtained when obtaining measurements for the biparietal diameter?
   a. Longitudinal
   b. Transverse
   c. Coronal

4. Which anatomic landmarks should be visualized along with the thalami when obtaining the biparietal diameter?
   a. Cavum septum pellucidi
   b. Cerebellar hemispheres
   c. Third ventricle

5. Where should the calipers be placed on the fetal skull for the biparietal diameter measurement?
   a. From outer to outer
   b. From inner to outer
   c. From outer to inner

6. Why is the head circumference more precise than the biparietal diameter in determining fetal age?
   a. The measurement is not shape dependent.
   b. It has a smaller margin of error.
   c. It incorporates the cephalic index.

7. When is the femur length most accurate in determining fetal growth?
   a. 15 to 32 weeks
   b. 12 to 28 weeks
   c. 24 to 36 weeks

8. In which view should the femur be measured?
   a. Caudal
   b. Transverse
   c. Longitudinal

9. What is the proper view for measuring the femur?
   a. The longest measurement of the femur excluding the diaphysis
   b. The longest measurement of the femur including the diaphysis
   c. The longest measurement of the femur with or without the epiphysis

10. After what gestational age does the epiphysis change from hypoechoic to hyperechoic?
    a. 13 weeks
    b. 28 weeks
    c. 32 weeks

11. Why is the femur closer to the transducer rather than farther from the transducer used for measurements of the femur?
    a. The femur farther from the transducer can display posterior shadowing, leading to deviant measurements.
    b. The femur closer to the transducer is less likely to move, which would make measurements more difficult to obtain.
    c. The femur farther from the transducer can make distinctions between epiphysis and diaphysis difficult to differentiate.

12. How should the transducer be placed on the maternal abdomen to obtain the fetal abdominal circumference?
    a. Image the fetus in a horizontal axis; turn the transducer into a transverse position
    b. Image the fetus in a longitudinal axis; turn the transducer into a transverse position
    c. Image the fetus in a longitudinal axis; turn the transducer into a coronal position

13. Which fetal parameter(s) does the abdominal circumference (AC) evaluate?
    a. Fetal growth alone
    b. Fetal growth and fetal weight
    c. Fetal growth and fetal age

14. Which fetal anatomic landmarks must be visualized to obtain the most accurate AC measurement?
    a. The kidneys and the umbilical vein joining the portal vein
    b. The stomach, the umbilical vein joining the portal vein, and the kidneys
    c. The stomach and the umbilical vein joining the portal vein

15. Where are the calipers placed for AC measurement?
    a. One caliper is placed on the outside of the anterior skin edge of the abdomen and the other caliper on the outside skin edge of the posterior spine.
    b. One caliper is placed on any portion of the anterior and posterior skin edges, as long as it includes the skin edge.

c. One caliper is placed on the inside of the anterior skin edge of the abdomen and the other caliper on the outside skin edge of the posterior spine.

16. When should comparative scans be scheduled if a fetus is being evaluated for a growth concern?
    a. Every 2 weeks
    b. Every 3 weeks
    c. Every week

17. What is the error rate for fetal weight predictions?
    a. ±15%
    b. ±25%
    c. ±5%

18. What is included in a standard ultrasound examination performed after 18 weeks' gestation that may be beyond the advanced practitioner's scope of practice?
    a. Elements of a fetal anatomic screen are done after 18 weeks' gestation.
    b. Doppler flow studies
    c. Maternal cervical length

19. What is the appearance of placental tissue toward the end of the third trimester?
    a. Echogenic focal thickening in the cotyledons
    b. Homogenous appearance within the cotyledons
    c. Hyperechoic lines of calcification outlining the cotyledons

20. What must be visualized to rule out a placenta previa beside the lower edge of the placenta?
    a. Internal cervical os
    b. Lower uterine segment
    c. Fetal presenting part

21. Which technical factors can mimic placenta previa?
    a. Insufficient ultrasound gel between skin and transducer
    b. Overall or total gain compensation set too low
    c. Focal uterine contractions or an overly distended bladder

22. Which sonographic findings might be present with a morbidly adherent placenta?
    a. A retroplacental complex that is a 1- to 2-cm hypoechoic band
    b. Loss of decidual interface between the placenta and the endometrium
    c. A "Swiss cheese" appearance on color Doppler

23. Upon what is the sonographic appearance of an abruption dependent?
    a. The "age" of the abruption
    b. The placental "age"
    c. The amount of bleeding

24. Which placental deviation from normal can appear as two placentas?
    a. A succenturiate or bilobed placenta
    b. A circumvallate placenta
    c. A placenta previa

25. What is the sonographic appearance of placental lakes?
    a. Anechoic
    b. Hyperechoic
    c. Hypoechoic

26. At what gestational age can cervical length can be reliably measured because the lower uterine segment and the cervix can be differentiated?
    a. 14 weeks
    b. 18 weeks
    c. 24 weeks

27. In what order do cervical shortening and dilation occur?
    a. From the external os at the cervical end toward the internal os at the uterine end
    b. From the inner os of the cervix at the uterine end toward the external os at the vaginal end
    c. At either end of the cervix

28. Which 3- to 9-MHz ultrasound probe is recommended for cervical length measurements?
    a. Transabdominal
    b. Translabial
    c. Transvaginal

29. Why is a generous amount of gel applied on both the inside and the outside of the transvaginal probe cover?
   a. To reduce probe cover friction that can obliterate the image
   b. To ease in the insertion of the TV probe
   c. To avoid air bubbles that will prevent the transmission of the sound waves and obscure the image

30. How is the cervical length measured if the cervical canal is curved?
   a. Trace the canal length.
   b. Measure it in two or more separate pieces and take the average.
   c. Release the transducer pressure to improve the image.

31. Which cervical length measurement should be reported after obtaining three total measurements?
   a. The shortest of the three measurements
   b. The average of the three measurements
   c. The longest of the three measurements

32. What is the significance of the sonographic visualization of funneling of the cervix as a predictor of preterm labor?
   a. It precedes dilation and cannot be palpated by an examining finger.
   b. It indicates impending spontaneous rupture of membranes.
   c. It is more common in breech presentations.

33. How is cervical length measured if funneling is present?
   a. From the lower uterine segment to the external os (the "open" length)
   b. From the onset of the funneling to the external os (the "closed" length)
   c. From the estimate of where the internal os is and the external os (the total length)

References

American College of Obstetricians and Gynecologists (ACOG). (2008). *Use of progesterone to reduce preterm birth.* ACOG Committee Opinion No. 419. Washington, DC: Author.

American College of Obstetricians and Gynecologists (ACOG). (2016a). *Prediction and prevention of preterm birth.* Technical Bulletin No. 130. Washington, DC: Author.

American College of Obstetricians and Gynecologists (ACOG). (2016b). *Ultrasound in pregnancy.* Technical Bulletin No. 175. Washington, DC: Author.

American College of Obstetricians and Gynecologists (ACOG). (2016c). Fetal macrosomia. Practice Bulletin No. 173. *Obstetrics and Gynecology, 128*, e195–e209.

American College of Obstetricians and Gynecologist (ACOG). (2017). Placenta accreta. Committee Opinion No. 529, Reaffirmed 2017. Retrieved from https://www.acog.org/Clinical-Guidance-and-Publications/Committee-Opinions/Committee-on-Obstetric-Practice/Placenta-Accreta

American College of Radiology. (2007). ACR practice guidelines for the performance of obstetrical ultrasound. In: *ACR practice guidelines and technical standards, 2007* (pp. 1025–1033). Reston, VA: Author.

American Institute of Ultrasound in Medicine (AIUM) (2018). AIUM-ACR-ACOG-SMFM-DRU Practice parameter for the performance of standard diagnostic obstetric ultrasound exams. Retrieved from: https://www.aium.org/resources/guidelines/obstetric.pdf

Ben-Haroush, A., Yogev, Y., Bar, J., Mashiach, R., Kaplan, B., Hod, M., & Meizner, I. (2004). Accuracy of sonographically estimated fetal weight in 840 women with different pregnancy complications prior to induction of labor. *Ultrasound in Obstetrics & Gynecology, 23*(2), 172–176.

Berghella, V. (2009). Novel developments on cervical length screening and progesterone for preventing preterm birth. *British Journal of Obstetrics and Gynecology, 116*(2), 182–187.

Berghella, V., & Khalifeh, A. (2018). Ultrasound evaluation of the gravid cervix. In P. W. Callen (Ed.), *Ultrasonography in obstetrics and gynecology* (6th ed., pp. 653–673) Philadelphia, PA: Elsevier.

Berghella, V., Talucci, M., & Desai, A. (2003). Does transvaginal sonographic measurement of cervical length before 14 weeks predict preterm delivery in high-risk pregnancies? *Ultrasound in Obstetrics & Gynecology, 21*(2), 140–144.

Berghella, V., Tolosa, J. E., Kuhlman, K. A., Weiner, S., Bolognese, R. J., & Wapner, R. J. (1997). Cervical ultrasonography compared to manual examination as a predictor of preterm delivery. *American Journal of Obstetrics and Gynecology, 177*, 723–730.

Cahill, A., Obido, A., Caughey, A., Stamilio, D. N., Hassan, S. S., Macones, G. A., & Romero, R. (2010). Universal cervical length screening and treatment with vaginal progesterone to prevent preterm birth: A decision and economic analysis. *American Journal of Obstetrics and Gynecology, 202*(6), 548.e1–548.e8. doi: 10.1016/j.ajog.2009.12.005

Campbell, S. (2011). Universal cervical-length and vaginal progesterone prevents early preterm births, reduces neonatal morbidity and is cost saving: Doing nothing is no longer an option. *Ultrasound in Obstetrics & Gynecology, 38*, 1–9.

Cawyer, C., Anderson, S., Szychowski, J., Neely, C., & Owen, J. (2018). Estimated gestational age with sonography. *Journal of Ultrasound in Medicine, 37*, 677–681.

Cervical Length Education and Review (CLEAR). (2018). Cervix measurement criteria. Retrieved from https://clear.perinatalquality.org/wfImageCriteria.aspx

Chory, M., Schnettler, W., March, M., Hacker, M., Modest, A., & Rodriguez, D. (2016). ACES: Accurate cervical evaluation with sonography. *Journal of Ultrasound in Medicine, 35,* 25–28.

Cicero, S., Skentou, C., Souka, A., & Nicolaides, K. H. (2001). Cervical length at 22–24 weeks of gestation: Comparison of transvaginal and transperineal–translabial ultrasonography. *Ultrasound in Obstetrics & Gynecology, 17*(4), 335–340.

Crane, J. M., & Hutchens, D. (2008). Transvaginal sonographic measurement of cervical length to predict preterm birth in asymptomatic women at increased risk: A systemic review. *Ultrasound in Obstetrics & Gynecology, 31*(5), 579–587.

Debbs, R. H., & Chen, J. (2009). Contemporary use of cerclage in pregnancy. *Clinical Obstetrics and Gynecology, 52,* 597–610.

Durfee, S. M., Frates, M., Luong, A., & Benson, C. B. (2005). The sonographic and color Doppler features of retained products of conception. *Journal of Ultrasound in Medicine, 24,* 1181–1186.

Faschingbauer, F., Dammer, U., Raabe, E., Kehl, S., Schmid, M., Schild, R., Beckmann, M., & Mayr, A. (2016). A new sonographic weight estimation formula for small-for-gestational-age fetuses. *Journal of Ultrasound in Medicine, 35,* 1713–1724.

Francois, K., Mayer, S., Harris, C., & Perlow, J. H. (2003). Association of vasa previa at delivery with a history of second-trimester placenta previa. *Journal of Reproductive Medicine, 48*(10), 771–774.

Ghi, T., Cariello, L., Rizzo, L., Ferrazzi, E., Periti, E., Prefumo, F., ... Rizzo, G., and the Società Italiana di Ecografia Ostetrica e Ginecologica Working Group on Fetal Biometric Charts. (2016). Customized fetal growth charts for parents' characteristics, race, and parity by quantile regression analysis. *Journal of Ultrasound in Medicine, 35,* 83–92.

Gramellini, D., Fieni, S., Molina, E., Beretta, R., & Vadora, E. (2002). Transvaginal sonographic cervical length changes during normal pregnancy. *Journal of Ultrasound in Medicine, 21*(3), 227–232.

Grobman, W., Lai, Y., Iams, J., Reddy, U., Mercer, B., Saade, G., ... Caritis, S. (2016). Prediction of spontaneous preterm birth among nulliparous women with a short cervix. *Journal of Ultrasound in Medicine, 35,* 1293–1297.

Hacking, C., & Radswiki, E. (2018). Placental abruption. Retrieved from https://radiopaedia.org/articles/placental-abruption

Hadlock, F. P., & Deter, R. L. (1982). Fetal biparietal diameter: A critical reevaluation of the relation to menstrual age by means of real-time ultrasound. *Journal of Ultrasound in Medicine, 1*(3), 97–104.

Hadlock, F. P., Deter, R. L., Harrist, R. B., & Park, S. K. (1982a). Fetal head circumference: Relation to menstrual age. *American Journal of Roentgenology, 138*(4), 649–653.

Hadlock, F. P., Deter, R. L., Harrist, R. B., & Park, S. K. (1982b). Fetal abdominal circumference as a predictor of menstrual age. *American Journal of Roentgenology, 139*(2), 367–370.

Hadlock, F. P., Harrist, R. B., Deter, R. L., & Park, S. K. (1982). Femur length as a predictor of menstrual age: Sonographically measured. *American Journal of Roentgenology, 138*(5), 875–878.

Harper, L. M., Roehl, K. A., Tuuli, M. G., Odibo, A. O., & Cahill, A. G. (2013). Sonographic accuracy of estimated fetal weight in twins. *Journal of Ultrasound in Medicine, 32,* 625–630.

Hassan, S., Romero, R., Vidyadhari, D., Fusey, S., Baxter, J. K., Khandelwal, M., ... Creasy, G. W. (2011). Vaginal progesterone reduces the rate of preterm birth in women with a sonographic short cervix: A multicenter, randomized, double-blind, placebo-controlled trial. *Ultrasound in Obstetrics & Gynecology, 38,* 18–31.

Hediger, M., Fuchs, K., Grantz, K., Grewal, J., Kim, S., Gore-Langton, R., ... Albert, P. (2016). Ultrasound quality assurance for singletons in the National Institute of Child Health and Human Development fetal growth studies. *Journal of Ultrasound in Medicine, 35,* 1725–1733.

Johnson, P. and Kutz A. (2018). Placenta previa. Retrieved from: https://sonoworld.com/CaseDetails/Placenta_previa.aspx?ModuleCategoryId=229

Kamaya, A., Petrovitch, I., Chen, B., Frederick, C. E., & Jeffrey, R. B. (2009). Retained products of conception: Spectrum of color Doppler findings. *Journal of Ultrasound in Medicine, 28,* 1031–1041.

Kiserud, T., Piaggio, G., Carroli, G., Widmer, M., Carvalho, J., Jensen, L. N., ... Platt, L. D. (2017). The World Health Organization fetal growth charts: A multinational longitudinal study of ultrasound biometric measurements and estimated fetal weight. *PLoS Med, 14*(1), e1002220. doi:10.1371/journal.pmed.1002220

Kulkarni, A., Powel, J., Aziz, M., Shah, L., Lashley, S., Benito, C., & Oyelese, Y. (2018). Vasa previa: Prenatal diagnosis and outcomes. *Journal of Ultrasound in Medicine, 37,* 1017–1024.

Kurmananvicius, J., Burkhardt, T., Wisser, J., & Huch, R. (2004). Ultrasonographic fetal weight estimation: Accuracy of formulas and accuracy of examiners by birth weight from 500–5,000 g. *Journal of Perinatal Medicine, 32*(2), 155–161.

Melamed, N., Meisner, I., Mashiach, R., Wiznitzer, A., Glezerman, M, & Yogey, Y.(2013). Fetal sex and intrauterine growth patterns. *Journal of Ultrasound in Medicine, 32,* 35–43

Melamed, N., Ryan, G., Windrim, R., Toi, A., & Kingdom, J. (2016). Choice of formula and accuracy of fetal weight estimation in small-for-gestational-age fetuses. *Journal of Ultrasound in Medicine, 35,* 71–82.

Mercer, B. M., Goldenberg, R. L., Das, A., Moawad, A. H., Iams, J. D., Meis, P. J., ... Roberts, J. (1996). The preterm prediction study: A clinical risk assessment system. *American Journal of Obstetrics and Gynecology, 174*(6), 1885–1893.

Moore, L. E., & Gonzalez, I. (2008). Placenta percreta with bladder invasion diagnosed with sonography: Images and clinical correlation. *Journal of Diagnostic Medical Sonography, 24,* 238–241.

Ness, A., Visintine, J., Ricci, E., & Berghella, V. (2007). Does knowledge of cervical length and fetal fibronectin affect management of women with threatened preterm labor?

A randomized trial. *American Journal of Obstetrics and Gynecology, 197*(4), 426.e1–426.e7.

O'Brien, J., & Sheehan, K. (2001). Prenatal diagnosis of a velamentous cord insertion associated with vasa previa. *Journal of Diagnostic Medical Sonography, 17,* 94–98.

Reddy, U., Abuhamad, A., Levine, D., & Saade, G. R. (2014). Fetal imaging: Executive summary of a joint Eunice Kennedy Shriver National Institute of Child Health and Human Development, Society for Maternal–Fetal Medicine, American Institute of Ultrasound in Medicine, American College of Obstetricians and Gynecologists, American College of Radiology, Society for Pediatric Radiology, and Society of Radiologists in Ultrasound Fetal Imaging workshop. *Journal of Ultrasound in Medicine, 33,* 745–757.

Rosati, P., & Guariglia, L. (2000). Clinical significance of placenta previa detected at early routine transvaginal scan. *Journal of Ultrasound in Medicine, 19,* 581–585.

Rust, O. A., Atlas, R. O., Kimmel, S., Roberts, W. E., & Hess, L. W. (2005). Does the presence of a funnel increase the risk of adverse perinatal outcome in a patient with a short cervix? *American Journal of Obstetrics and Gynecology, 192*(4), 1060–1066.

Sanin-Blair, J., Palacia, M., Delgado, J., Figueras, F., Coll, O., Cabero, L., . . . Gratacos E. (2004). Impact of ultrasound cervical length assessment on duration of hospital stay in the clinical management of threatened preterm labor. *Ultrasound in Obstetrics & Gynecology, 24*(7), 756–760

Saul, L., Kurtzman, T., Hagemann, C., Ghamsary, M., & Wing, D. (2008). Is transabdominal sonography of the cervix after voiding a reliable method of cervical length assessment? *Journal of Ultrasound in Medicine, 27,* 1305–1311.

Schild, R. L., Sachs, C., Fimmers, R., Gembruch, U., & Hansmann, M. (2004). Sex-specific fetal weight prediction by ultrasound. *Ultrasound in Obstetrics & Gynecology, 23*(1), 30–35.

Schwarzler, P., Bland, J. M., Holden, D., Campbell, S. & Ville, Y. (2004). Sex-specific antenatal reference growth charts for uncomplicated singleton pregnancies at 15–40 weeks of gestation. *Ultrasound in Obstetrics & Gynecology, 23*(1), 23–29.

Shinde, G. R., Vaswani, B. P., Patange, R. P., Laddad, M. M., & Bhosale, R. B. (2016). Diagnostic performance of ultrasonography for detection of abruption and its clinical correlation and maternal and foetal outcome. *Journal of Clinical and Diagnostic Research, 10*(8), QC04-7. doi: 10.7860 /JCDR/2016/19247.8288

Smith, G. C., Celik, E., To, M., Khouri, M., & Nicolaides, K. H. (2008). Cervical length at mid-pregnancy and the risk of primary cesarean delivery. *New England Journal of Medicine, 358*(13), 1346–1353.

Smith, N. C., & Smith, P. M. (2003). *Obstetric ultrasound made easy.* Edinburgh, UK: Churchill Livingstone.

Society for Maternal-Fetal Medicine (SMFM) (2015). Consult Series #37: Diagnosis and management of vasa previa. Society of Maternal-Fetal (SMFM) Publications Committee; Rachel G. Sinkey, MD; Anthony O. Odibo, MD, MSCE; Jodi S. Dashe, MD. Retrieved from https://www.ajog.org/article /S0002-9378(15)00897-2/pdf

Society for Maternal-Fetal Medicine (SMFM) (2016). Consult Series I #40: The role of routine cervical length screening in selected high- and low-risk women for preterm birth prevention. Society for Maternal-Fetal Medicine (SMFM); Jennifer McIntosh, MD; Helen Feltovich, MD; Vincenzo Berghella, MD; Tracy Manuck, MD; retrieved from: https:// www.ajog.org/article/S0002-9378(16)30112-0/pdf

Taylor, B. K. (2011). Sonographic assessment of cervical length and the risk of preterm birth. *Journal of Obstetric, Gynecologic, & Neonatal Nursing, 40*(5), 617–631.

Thompson, M. O., Vines, S. K., Aquilina, J., Wathen, N. C., & Harrington, K. (2002). Are placental lakes of any clinical significance? *Placenta, 23*(8–9), 685–690.

Valent, A., Newman, T., Kritzer, S., Magner, K., & Warshak, C. (2017). Accuracy of sonographically estimated fetal weight near delivery in pregnancies complicated with diabetes mellitus. *Journal of Ultrasound in Medicine, 36,* 593–599.

Williams, P. L., Laifer-Narin, S. L., & Ragavendra, N. (2003). US of abnormal uterine bleeding. *Radiographics, 23*(3), 703–718.

Yost, N. P., Bloom, S. L., Twickler, D. M., & Leveno, K. J. (1999). Pitfalls in ultrasonic cervical length measurement for predicting preterm birth. *Obstetrics and Gynecology, 93*(4), 510–516.

CHAPTER 6

Ultrasound Evaluation of Fetal Well-Being

▶ Introduction

The most common antepartum evaluation test of fetal well-being is the nonstress test (NST), which utilizes the electronic fetal monitor. In most cases, when the NST is not reassuring of fetal well-being, a second test is performed, the biophysical profile, using ultrasound. The BPP is generally performed following a nonreactive NST, although, in some cases, it is the first line of antepartum testing employed in either its full application or with its modified use (the modified BPP). This chapter describes each component of the sonographic portion of the BPP.

▶ The Biophysical Profile

The BPP was developed in 1980 by Manning and associates (1981). It combines traditional electronic fetal monitoring (EFM) with a sonographic fetal evaluation. Manning et al. (1981) viewed this technique as an intrauterine physical examination of the fetus, comparable to Apgar scoring in the neonate. Nearly 40 years after its introduction, the BPP remains one of the key tools in the prenatal assessment of fetal well-being.

The underlying premise of the BPP is the relationship between oxygen and the central nervous system (CNS) response as observed by ultrasound. As the fetal CNS matures with advancing gestational age, fetal behavior develops in a specific order. Fetal tone (FT) begins to be evident by ultrasound around 7½ to 8 weeks' gestation, followed by fetal movement (FM) beginning around 9 weeks' gestation. Fetal breathing (FB) becomes regular at 20 to 21 weeks' gestation, followed by development of fetal heart rate (FHR) control (i.e., the ability to accelerate and decelerate) at the end of the second trimester or beginning of the third trimester.

With an insidious or chronic loss of fetal oxygenation, the fetus begins to lose these same behaviors, but in the *opposite* order in which they developed. So, in the event of chronic oxygen deprivation, initially there will be the loss of fetal heart reactivity, followed by a decrease or loss of fetal breathing movements (FBM). If the oxygen deprivation continues, a decrease in amniotic fluid will occur. Ultimately, there will be a loss of FM with, finally, the loss of FT (Manning et al., 1981). Although factors other than deoxygenation may cause a change in some or all of these behaviors, these parameters, when present, are highly predictive of fetal oxygenation and fetal well-being; thus, they are used as the basis of the BPP. Knowledge of the five parameters, their progressive emergence throughout gestational age, and the pattern of decline seen with increasing hypoxia can provide invaluable information regarding the oxygenation status of the fetus.

The BPP has a very low false-negative rate, indicating that a score of 8/10 or 10/10 is highly predictive of adequate fetal oxygenation and the absence of fetal metabolic acidemia. However, each BPP parameter by itself has a high false-positive rate. For example, absence of fetal breathing alone may be the result of sleep cycles, medication affects, or some unknown cause other than deoxygenation. The false-positive rate can be greatly reduced when the parameters are combined. The specific criteria for each parameter were defined by Manning using a scoring system of 2 points if the parameter is present and 0 if it is absent (**TABLE 6-1**) (Manning et al., 1981; Manning et al., 1987). There is no partial score. This examination is still considered a highly reliable method for fetal

evaluation (American College of Obstetricians and Gynecologists [ACOG], 2016).

In 1983, Vintzileos et al. (1983) proposed a modification to Manning's scoring system. In addition to Manning's five parameters, they introduced a sixth parameter: placental grading based on the degree of maturation of the placenta. A mature placenta is given the highest score, and the immature placenta a low score. Additionally, the change to the scoring system for each parameter included adding a middle point value option, a score of 1, that accounted for the observation of partial fetal behaviors, borderline amniotic fluid levels, or the inability to grade the placenta (**TABLE 6-2**) (Vintzileos et al., 1983).

Both forms of BPPs have similar neonatal outcome predictive value. However, the Manning BPP is utilized nearly universally in the United States. Whichever BPP point system is selected for use in a particular healthcare setting, its application should be clarified and established in a protocol. Potentially, clinical management could be adversely impacted if only a raw score is reported. For instance, a loss

TABLE 6-1 Manning Biophysical Profile Scoring System

Criterion	Score	
	2	0
Fetal tone	One episode of flexion/extension of fetal spine, limbs, or hand	Extremities in extension
Fetal movement	Three gross body movements including rolling	Two or fewer episodes of fetal movement
Fetal breathing	30 seconds of continuous breathing	Absence of respiratory effort
Nonstress test (NST)	Two accelerations 15 bpm × 15 seconds within 20 minutes	Nonreactive NST
Amniotic fluid volume (AFV)	Largest fluid pocket > 2 cm vertically (preferred) or amniotic fluid index (AFI) > 5 cm	Largest fluid pocket < 2 cm vertically or AFI < 5 cm

Modified from ACOG (2016), Manning et al. (1981).

TABLE 6-2 Vintzileos Biophysical Scoring System

Criterion	Score		
	2	**1**	**0**
Fetal tone	One episode of flexion/extension of extremity *and* one episode of spine extension/flexion	One episode of flexion/extension of extremity *or* one episode of spine extension/flexion	Extremities in extension
Fetal movement	At least three episodes of gross body movements within 30 minutes	One or two gross body movements within 30 minutes	Absence of gross body movements within 30 minutes
Fetal breathing	At least one episode of fetal breathing sustained for minimum of 60 seconds during 30 minutes	At least one episode of fetal breathing sustained for 30–60 seconds during 30 minutes	No fetal breathing or breathing lasting less than 30 seconds
Nonstress test (NST)	At least five or more 15 bpm × 15 seconds accelerations associated with fetal movement in a 20-minute time frame	Two to four 15 bpm × 15 seconds accelerations associated with fetal movement in a 20-minute time frame	Fewer than one 15 bpm × 15 seconds acceleration associated with fetal movement in a 20-minute time frame
Amniotic fluid volume	> 2 cm vertical pocket	A vertical pocket that measures < 2 cm but > 1 cm	Crowding of fetal small parts with < 1 cm vertical fluid pocket
Placental grading	Score 0, 1, or 2	Placenta posterior and difficult to grade	Score 3

Data from Vintzileos, A. M., Campbell, W. A., Ingardia, C. J., & Nochimson, D. (1983). The biophysical profile and its predictive value. Obstetrics and Gynecology, 62(2), 271–278.

of 2 points for oligohydramnios and 2 points for absence of FM would give a score of 8 (out of 12) on the Vintzileos scale and a 6 (out of 10) on the Manning scale. In this example, the raw score of 8 on the Vintzileos scale would be falsely reassuring if it is believed to be based on the Manning criteria. It is imperative to express the score with both the numerator and the denominator (8/12 or 8/10) so that the test may be interpreted correctly. For the purposes of this chapter, the BPP parameters and scoring system presented will be based on the Manning 10-point criteria.

▶ Biophysical Profile Parameters

Each of the parameters of the biophysical profile is described in this section:

- Fetal heart reactivity (NST)
- Fetal tone
- Fetal movement
- Fetal breathing activity
- Amniotic fluid volume (AFV)

Fetal Heart Reactivity

Fetal heart reactivity is determined by performing an NST that is interpreted as either reactive or nonreactive. Although the criteria for a reactive pattern may vary among institutions, the most commonly accepted criterion for a reactive NST is the presence of two accelerations within 20 minutes of testing. Each acceleration must last for 15 seconds, with a peak amplitude of 15 beats per minute (bpm) above the baseline FHR (**FIGURE 6-1**). The NST is considered nonreactive when it fails to meet the stated criteria for a reactive NST (i.e., fails to demonstrate adequate fetal heart rate accelerations; see **FIGURE 6-2**). An additional 20 minutes can be used to evaluate reactivity since it is well established that fetal sleep–wake cycles may be up to 40 minutes in length (ACOG, 2016; Finberg, Kurtz, Johnson, & Wapner, 1990; Vintzileos et al., 1983).

A reactive NST is considered one of the best predictors of fetal well-being and the absence of fetal metabolic acidemia. However, a nonreactive NST has a false positive rate of 40% to 80%, meaning that the cause of the nonreactivity may be something other than hypoxia. Therefore, a nonreactive NST needs to be followed by another form of fetal evaluation to differentiate the hypoxic fetus from the nonhypoxic fetus. The BPP is the most commonly used follow-up test (ACOG, 2016; Finberg et al., 1990).

Fetal Tone

FT is the first of the five parameters to develop during fetal CNS maturation. It is defined as the observer witnessing at least one of the following fetal activities: limb extension with return to flexion, flexion/extension of the spine, or opening and closing of the hand.

Fetal Movement

FM is defined as the observation of flexion and extension of extremities and/or rolling motions of the fetal trunk. Three distinct episodes of FM are required to achieve a full score. Simultaneous movement of more than one body part is counted as a single movement, just as are isolated limb movements.

Fetal Breathing Movements

FBM increases in frequency and duration with advancing gestational age. Ultrasound observation

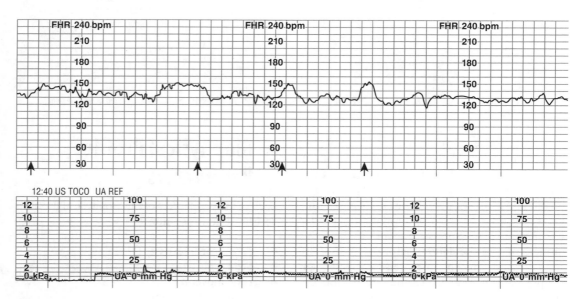

FIGURE 6-1 Reactive nonstress test (NST).

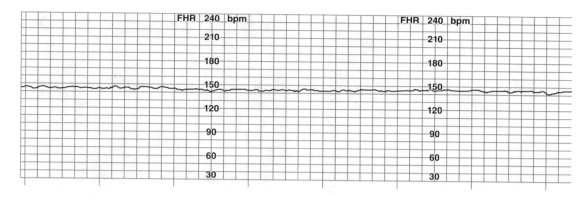

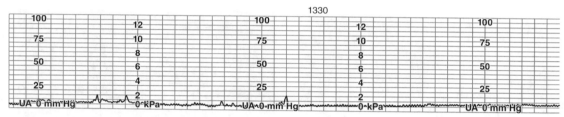

FIGURE 6-2 Nonreactive nonstress test (NST).

reveals the presence of diaphragmatic and chest wall excursion, which is often best visualized at the level of the diaphragm (**FIGURE 6-3**, A and B). A minimum of 30 seconds of *continuous* fetal breathing is required. The presence or absence of fetal breathing as a reliable indicator of well-being must be evaluated carefully. It is known that FBMs are sporadic, vary with gestational age, exhibit diurnal variations, and are often absent in the presence of labor. FBMs are known to be reduced in women who have been fasting (Mirghani, Weerasinghe, Ezimokhai, & Smith, 2003) and following glucocorticosteroid administration (Jackson, Kleeman, Doerzbacher, & Lambers, 2003).

Amniotic Fluid Volume

Amniotic fluid may be measured either by the deepest pocket method or by the amniotic fluid index (AFI) for the BPP, although more recent studies suggest the single deepest pocket has a higher predictive value for oligohydramnios (ACOG, 2016). Regardless of the techniques being used,

the fluid measured should be free of fetal parts or umbilical cord. AFV becomes stable between 26 and 38 weeks, after which a normal gradual decline may be observed. At term, normal AFV is defined as the single deepest vertical pocket of amniotic fluid of 2 cm or more or an AFI (sum of fluid measurements in four quadrants) of more than 5 cm.

Reduced amniotic fluid may be the result of normal fluid decline as gestation increases or rupture of membranes; however, it may be an indicator of chronic fetal compromise leading to reduced fetal renal profusion and reduced urinary output (Magann, Sandlin, & Ounpraseuth, 2011; Shank et al., 2011). Although it is possible that pockets of amniotic fluid may be missed in obese women, Blitz and colleagues (2018) found that increasing maternal body mass index (BMI) is not associated with oligohydramnios in late gestations. Regardless of the cause, a significantly reduced AFV is a risk for the pregnancy because it may contribute to cord compression, poor perinatal outcome, and possibly fetal death.

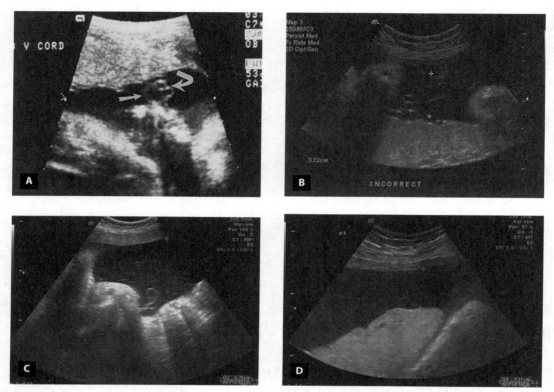

FIGURE 6-3 A. Single-pocket fluid measurement at the deepest pocket (colored arrow), excluding the umbilical cord (between white arrows). **B.** Single-pocket fluid measurement performed *incorrectly* (between cursors)—measurement should also include the areas of the umbilical cord indicated by the arrow. **C.** Single-pocket fluid measurement performed correctly by omitting the area of the umbilical cord indicated by the arrow. **D.** Correct measurement of the single fluid pocket, between the cursors.

Current data show that, regardless of the method used to identify oligohydramnios (subjective, AFI, or deepest pocket), overdiagnosis of oligohydramnios is occurring. Overdiagnosis often leads to unnecessary inductions and may contribute to increased neonatal morbidity and mortality without demonstrating improvement in perinatal outcomes (ACOG, 2016; Driggers, Holcroft, Blakemore, & Graham, 2004; Magann et al., 2004; Magann et al., 2011; Morris, 2004 et al.; Nabhan & Abdelmoula, 2012; Phelan et al., 1987).

As a result of these concerns about overdiagnosis, ACOG has defined oligohydramnios based on randomized controlled trials (RCTs) as a single deepest vertical pocket of amniotic fluid of 2 cm or less (not containing the umbilical cord or fetal extremities) and supports the use of the deepest vertical pocket of amniotic fluid to diagnose oligohydramnios (2016).

Sonographic Techniques for Amniotic Fluid Assessment

Using the single-pocket method, at least one pocket of amniotic fluid that is 2 cm or greater in vertical dimension is identified. Areas with umbilical cord visible should not be measured. Measuring up to the edge of the cord is acceptable (Figure 6-3, A and C). An AFV of more than 2 cm receives 2 points on the Manning BPP scoring system and is considered normal fluid volume (Figure 6-3D).

The AFI is obtained by measuring the largest pocket of fluid in each of the four quadrants of the uterus (**FIGURE 6-4 , COLOR PLATES A, B, C**). The sum of

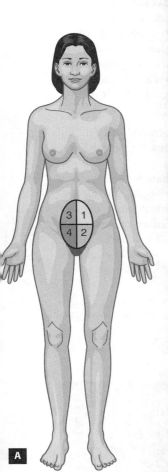

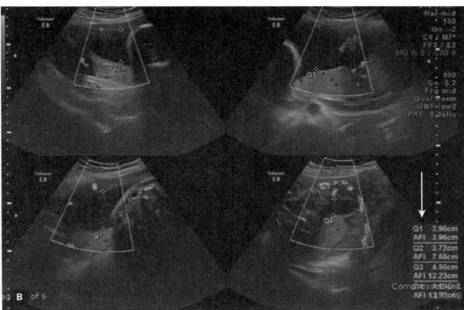

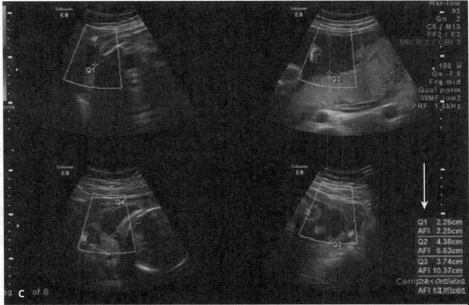

FIGURE 6-4 A. Dividing the maternal abdomen into four quadrants for measuring the amniotic fluid index (AFI). **B.** AFI with color flow Doppler identification of the umbilical cord in the pocket. The four individual quadrant measurements of amniotic fluid are between the "+" signs. Note each quadrant measurement at the large arrow, which has been generated by the ultrasound machine, along with the total of the four quadrants. The total AFI is in the lower-right corner (arrow). **C.** AFI with color flow Doppler of the umbilical cord, ensuring it is not included in the measurement.

the four quadrant measurements is the actual AFI. Serial AFI evaluations provide the clinician with a semiquantitative volume of fluid and the ability to assess overall changes with time and patient status. An AFI of 5 to 18 cm is considered normal at term. AFIs at or less than 5 cm may be diagnostic of oligohydramnios (**FIGURE 6-5**) and are associated with nonreactive NSTs, variable decelerations, meconium staining, and 5-minute Apgar scores of less than 7 (Phelan et al., 1987), as well as with an increase in operative delivery for suspected fetal compromise (ACOG, 2016).

Management Strategies for Oligohydramnios and Polyhydramnios

When oligohydramnios is diagnosed by AFI, medical intervention often follows in the form of an induction of labor or surgical intervention. However, amniotic fluid can increase with hydration and rest. In one study, women with normal amounts of amniotic fluid (AFI of 6 to 24 cm) were divided into two groups: (1) women undergoing maternal rest in the left lateral decubitus position with oral hydration and (2) women positioned in the left lateral decubitus position alone. The results showed

that the two groups had similar increases in AFV at 15 minutes post hydration/rest. However, after 30 minutes, the AFV increased more rapidly in the hydration group (Kahraman & Melek, 2013).

Another study examined maternal hydration and pregnancy outcomes when intravenous (IV) hydration was administered in response to isolated oligohydramnios. The results demonstrated that IV hydration improved the quantity of amniotic fluid in the oligohydramnios group (Patrelli et al., 2012).

Based on expert opinion, ACOG (2016) recommends the following:

- With otherwise uncomplicated isolated and persistent oligohydramnios, plan for delivery at 36–37 weeks' gestation.
- In pregnancies at less than 36 0/7 weeks of gestation with intact membranes and oligohydramnios, expectant management or delivery should be individualized based on gestational age and the maternal and fetal condition.
- If delivery is not undertaken, follow-up AFV measurements, NSTs, and fetal growth assessments are indicated.
- If the oligohydramnios results from fetal membrane rupture, follow-up AFV assessment often may be safely omitted.

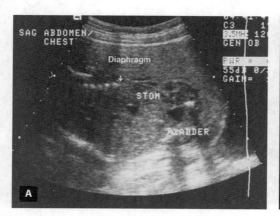 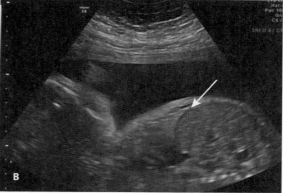

FIGURE 6-5 A. Oligohydramnios with no measurable fluid observed, with confirmation of urine in the bladder prior to treatment with amnioinfusion. Note how much more difficult it is to visualize the fetus when the acoustic window that the amniotic fluid normally provides is lacking. This is evident when comparing panels A and B. The anechoic vertical "stripe" is the diaphragm (small white arrow), which divides the abdominal contents from the chest. **B.** Normal fluid, with the fetal diaphragm also visible as an anechoic strip around the abdominal contents (at the arrow).

Doppler blood flow studies of the fetal–placental pair have further improved obstetric care and antepartum testing, particularly in the growth-restricted fetus. Currently, there is no evidence that umbilical artery Doppler velocimetry provides information about fetal well-being in the fetus with normal growth. Moreover, concurrent use of color Doppler with assessment of the AFV results in overdiagnosis of oligohydramnios (ACOG, 2016; Eden et al., 1988).

Polyhydramnios has been defined as an AFI of greater than 24 cm (**FIGURE 6-6**) (Magann et al., 2004) or a single pocket of greater than 8 cm (Reddy, Abuhamad, Levine, & Saade, 2014). Polyhydramnios is associated with numerous congenital anomalies, particularly those involving the gastrointestinal (GI) tract. It is also associated with maternal viral infections.

▶ Assessment and Scoring of the BPP

The maximum period of time for evaluating the ultrasound parameters of the BPP is 30 minutes, exclusive of the NST. The NST may be performed prior to or following the ultrasound portion of the procedure. As mentioned previously, assessment and scoring of the BPP depend on whether Manning's or Vintzileos's criteria are used. The main difference between the two scoring systems is that with Manning's system, the score is 2 or 0: Either the behavior is present or it is not. A partial point of 1 is not used. With Vintzileos's system, a partial score of 1 is given with partial demonstration of the behavior. A second difference is that Vintzileos's system includes a sixth parameter, placental grading, for which a score is given depending on placental maturity. A mature placenta shows sonographic demarcations of the placental cotyledons, indicating it is mature. The immature placenta has a sonographically smoother appearance (isoechogenic). It cannot be emphasized enough that obstetrical providers and advanced practitioners must know which assessment and scoring method is being utilized at the institution performing the BPP so that appropriate management based on the results can be instituted.

▶ Application and Management of BPP Results

The results of all antepartum fetal evaluations should be considered in conjunction with complete maternal–fetal history and clinical circumstances.

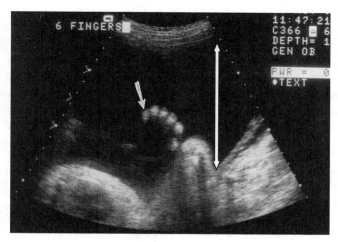

FIGURE 6-6 Polyhydramnios (only one pocket shown, with total fluid measurement of 36 cm). Also note the sixth digit at the small arrow.

TABLE 6-3	Application of Biophysical Profile Results Based on Manning's BPP	
BPP Score	**Interpretation**	**Recommended Management**
10	Non-asphyxiated fetus	No intervention. Repeat testing weekly or 2 times per week, depending on the indication.
8–10	Normal non-asphyxiated fetus	No fetal indications for intervention. Repeat per protocol.
8 or 10 with decreased fluid	Chronic fetal asphyxia suspected	Deliver.
6	Possible fetal asphyxia	<ul><li>Deliver if amniotic fluid volume (AFV) is abnormal at 36–37 weeks.</li><li>If normal fluid and more than 36 weeks' gestation with a favorable cervix, deliver.</li><li>If less than 36 weeks' gestation or immature lungs or an unfavorable cervix, repeat in 24 hours.</li><li>If the score on the repeat test is 6 or less, deliver. If the score on the repeat test is greater than 6, observe and repeat per protocol.</li></ul>
4	Probable asphyxia	Repeat testing same day. If the score on the repeat test is 6 or less, deliver. In pregnancies at less than 32 0/7 weeks' gestation, management should be individualized, and extended monitoring may be appropriate.
0–2	Almost certain asphyxia	Deliver.

Modified from ACOG (2016), Manning et al. (1981).

However, management recommendations of the raw scores in the BPP can be found in **TABLE 6-3**.

The BPP has also been used during labor to assess fetal well-being when the EFM strip was nonreassuring. It has been shown to predict the need for cesarean delivery (Kim et al., 2003).

▶ Modified Biophysical Profile

The "modified BPP" is a condensed version of the full BPP. It consists of an NST in conjunction with just the AFV assessment using either Phelan's four-quadrant AFI method (Kim et al., 2003; Rutherford, Phelan, Smith, & Jacobs, 1987) or the single-pocket measurement, which is recommended by ACOG (2016). The remaining parameters of the BPP (fetal breathing, movement, and tone) are not used. The rationale is that if accelerations of the FHR are present in response to maternal perception of FM during the NST, then FM exists and does not need to be directly observed by ultrasound. Additionally, the presence of FM indicates that fetal muscle tone is present.

The modified BPP consumes less time, as well as requires less extensive training and education of the person performing the biophysical profile. The only ultrasound skill required is in the measurement of amniotic fluid volume (AFV). However, there are theoretical risks to this if a nonsonographer is taught how to measure fluid, but is not fully educated in other principles of point-of-care (POC) ultrasound.

The modified BPP is used with both the low-risk and high-risk obstetric groups. A recent study has confirmed that the application of modified BPP in high-risk populations has the same outcome predictions as with the full BPP (Sowmya, Mudanur, Padmasri, & Lalitha, 2017).

▶ POC Biophysical Profile Procedure

Advanced practitioners (APs) who have obtained the appropriate didactic and clinical education in ultrasound may perform BPPs, fluid assessments, and Doppler studies (American College of Nurse-Midwives [ACNM], 2018; American Institute of Ultrasound in Medicine [AIUM], 2018; Association of Women's Health, Obstetric and Neonatal Nurses [AWHONN], 2016; Gegor, Paine, Costigan, & Johnson, 1994). Preparation with the recommended number of didactic hours and determination of clinical competency must be achieved.

The general technique for performing a BPP is to have the woman positioned supine with some lateral tilt to avoid supine hypotension. The clinician performing the BPP should be in a comfortable position because the test may involve holding the ultrasound transducer somewhat stationary for 30 minutes. The BPP parameters may be obtained in any order.

Once the fetal presentation and lie have been identified, the fetal torso and extremities are observed for movement, flexion, and extension. By holding the transducer in place, fetal movement and tone can be observed by watching the fetal part move in real time. For example, the spine may be visible and then move out of the field of view; this indicates FM. Specific to tone, however, both flexion and extension need to be visualized so as not to confuse them with fetal movement. The flexion/extension may be of the hand opening and closing, or the spine arching and returning to a neutral position. It could also be a leg kicking or the toes flexing and extending.

Observing for FBM can be more challenging. Many sonographers will begin by following the fetal spine in the transverse plane. Then, at the level of the heart, the transducer is turned into the sagittal plane, gaining a long axis of the chest and abdomen. It is at this level that the fetal diaphragm will be seen and FBMs observed as the abdominal wall expands and contracts. FBM may be seen in other planes as well, but the motion should not be mistaken for maternal abdominal wall movements.

At any point during the BPP when FBM is observed, it is advised to focus on the breathing motion until the full 30 seconds has passed. Other parameters may also be detected simultaneously; however, because FBM is intermittent and elusive, the sonographer should seize the opportunity.

▶ Other Indications for POC Amniotic Fluid Assessment

Prior to performing external cephalic version, the fetal status is evaluated with some combination of antepartum testing. In most situations, amniotic fluid is assessed prior to the attempt at version. The success rate of the version is directly related to the quantity of amniotic fluid (Kok et al., 2009).

In addition, when variable decelerations are present on the reactive NST, an amniotic fluid assessment should be performed to determine whether oligohydramnios is present. The reactive NST indicates the absence of fetal metabolic acidemia at the time of testing, but if variable decelerations become recurrent, fetal metabolic acidemia may develop. One of the most common causes of variable decelerations is oligohydramnios; thus, it is the underlying indication that warrants quantifying amniotic fluid under these circumstances.

▶ Summary

Interpretation and recommended follow-up based on the BPP results are presented in Table 6-3. However, it is imperative that management decisions not be based solely on the NST or BPP score. Such decisions could lead to unnecessary interventions or even adverse outcomes. Management decisions should be made after careful review of the patient's overall clinical picture.

In 2009, the participants at a Eunice Kennedy Shriver National Institute of Child Health and Human Development workshop, "Antenatal Testing: A Reevaluation," reviewed the literature on antepartum testing. Their overall conclusion was that there are gaps in the evidence "guiding the clinical application of most antepartum assessments commonly in use today" and that there is a need for further research. However, all antepartum tests that were reviewed (NST, CST, BPP, and modified BPP) showed very low false-negative rates (between 0.2% and 0.65%). Thus, if the test result is reassuring, it appears to be highly predictive of fetal well-being and the absence of fetal metabolic acidemia. However, if the test result is "positive," indicating possible fetal compromise, it may be poorly predictive. Depending on which test is used, between 35% and 90% of the neonates with "positive" test results are born without compromise (Signore, Freeman, & Sponge, 2009).

Generally, tests performed in combination (i.e., the NST and BPP) have shown the best outcome results. However, along with these tests comes an associated financial burden. The most common indication for antepartum fetal evaluation is postdates pregnancy, which affects a relatively large of number of women and, therefore, carries a relatively high cost. However, in many "postdates" cases, the dating of the pregnancy is inaccurate. Therefore, one of the most cost-effective methods for reducing the expense of antepartum evaluation of the postdates pregnancy can be accomplished by ensuring accurate dating of the pregnancy. The most predictive methods of pregnancy dating include the following (ACOG, 2016):

- Ultrasound dating performed at less than 20 weeks' gestation
- A minimum of 30 weeks since a positive serum or urine pregnancy test along with documented fetal heart tones for a minimum of 30 weeks by Doppler

The costs associated with antepartum testing have tremendous societal impact (Fonseca, Monga, & Silva, 2003). However, women who have late prenatal care and/or uncertain pregnancy dating must be tested when they reach 41 weeks regardless of how uncertain the dating criteria being utilized.

Study Questions

1. When does fetal tone begin to be visualized by ultrasound?
   a. Approximately 5 to 7 weeks
   b. Approximately 7½ to 8 weeks
   c. Approximately 8½ to 10 weeks

2. When does fetal movement begin to be visualized by ultrasound?
   a. Approximately 5 to 7 weeks
   b. Approximately 7½ to 8 weeks
   c. Approximately 8½ to 10 weeks

3. When does fetal breathing begin to be visualized by ultrasound?
   a. Approximately 20 to 21 weeks
   b. Approximately 22 to 24 weeks
   c. Approximately 25 to 27 weeks

4. When do fetal heart rate accelerations and decelerations begin to be apparent on the fetal monitor?
   a. At the end of the second trimester or the beginning of the third trimester
   b. Early in the second trimester
   c. Beginning in the third trimester

5. In what order will the fetus begin to lose these same behaviors when faced with an insidious or chronic loss of fetal oxygenation?
   a. In the same order in which they developed
   b. In any order depending on the cause of deoxygenation
   c. In the opposite order in which they developed

6. What can cause decreased amniotic fluid volume in the absence of ruptured membranes or fetal renal abnormalities?
   a. Increasing maternal body mass index
   b. Chronic fetal deoxygenation
   c. Shunting of oxygenated blood to the kidneys

7. How is fetal tone assessed on the biophysical profile (BPP)?
   a. The observer witnesses at least three episodes of limb extension with a return to flexion, flexion/extension of the spine, or the opening and closing of the hand.
   b. The observer witnesses at least one episode of limb extension with a return to flexion, flexion/extension of the spine, or the opening and closing of the hand.
   c. The observer witnesses at least two episodes of limb extension with return to flexion, flexion/extension of the spine, or the opening and closing of the hand.

8. How is fetal breathing assessed on the BPP?
   a. 30 cumulative seconds of fetal breathing observed over the 30 minutes of testing
   b. The presence of episodic fetal breathing throughout the duration of testing
   c. 30 seconds or longer of continuous fetal breathing observed

9. How is fetal movement assessed on the BPP?
   a. Three distinct episodes of flexion and extension of the extremities and/or rolling motions of the fetal trunk or isolated limb movements
   b. Two distinct episodes of flexion and extension of the extremities and/or rolling motions of the fetal trunk or isolated limb movements
   c. One distinct episodes of flexion and extension of the extremities and/or rolling motions of the fetal trunk or isolated limb movements

10. What is the definition of oligohydramnios when the single-pocket method is used?
    a. Less than a 5-cm vertical pocket
    b. Aggregate of four vertical pockets less than 5 cm
    c. Less than a 2-cm vertical pocket

11. Which tests have been noted to have a high false-positive rate in the diagnosis of oligohydramnios?
    a. AFI and Doppler flow
    b. Both AFV and AFI
    c. AFV alone

12. What is the most common fetal anatomic placement of the ultrasound transducer to view fetal breathing movements?
    a. Kidneys
    b. Lungs
    c. Diaphragm

References

American College of Nurse-Midwives (ACNM). (2018). *Position statement: Ultrasound for midwives.* Washington, DC: Author.

American College of Obstetricians and Gynecologists (ACOG). (2016a). *Induction of labor.* Technical Bulletin No. 107. Washington, DC: Author.

American College of Obstetricians and Gynecologists (ACOG). (2016b). Antepartum fetal surveillance. Practice Guideline No. 145. Washington, DC: Author.

American Institute of Ultrasound in Medicine (AIUM). (2018). AIUM practice parameter for the performance of limited obstetric ultrasound examinations by advanced clinical providers. Retrieved from https://www.aium.org/resources/guidelines/LimitedOB_Providers.pdf

Association of Women's Health, Obstetric and Neonatal Nurses (AWHONN). (2016). *Ultrasound examinations performed by nurses in obstetric, gynecologic and reproductive medicine settings.* Washington, DC: Author.

Blitz, M., Rockelson, B., Stork, L., Augustine, S., Greenberg, M., Sison, C., & Vohra, N. (2018). Maternal body mass index and amniotic fluid index in late gestation. *Journal of Ultrasound in Medicine, 37,* 561–568.

Driggers, R. W., Holcroft, C. J., Blakemore, K. J., & Graham, E. M. (2004). An amniotic fluid index < or =5 cm within 7 days of delivery in the third trimester is not associated with decreasing umbilical arterial pH and base excess. *Journal of Perinatology, 24*(2), 72–76.

Eden, R. D., Seifert, L. S., Kodack, L. D., Trofatter, L. D., Killam, A. P., & Gail, S. A. (1988). A modified biophysical profile for antenatal fetal surveillance: Part 1. *Obstetrics and Gynecology, 71*(3), 365–369.

Finberg, H. J., Kurtz, A. B., Johnson, R., & Wapner, R. (1990). The biophysical profile: A literature review and reassessment of its usefulness in the evaluation of fetal well-being. *Journal of Ultrasound in Medicine, 9*(10), 583–591.

Fonseca, L., Monga, M., & Silva, J. (2003). Postdates pregnancy in an indigent population: The financial burden. *American Journal of Obstetrics and Gynecology, 188*(5), 1214–1216.

Gegor, C., Paine, L. L., Costigan, K., & Johnson, T. R. B. (1994). Interpretation of biophysical profiles by nurses and physicians. *Journal of Obstetric, Gynecologic, & Neonatal Nursing, 23*(5), 114–119.

Jackson, J. R., Kleeman, S., Doerzbacher, M., & Lambers, D. S. (2003). The effect of glucocorticosteroid administration on fetal movements and biophysical profile scores in normal pregnancies. *Journal of Maternal–Fetal and Neonatal Medicine, 13*(1), 50–53.

Kahraman, U., & Melek, C. (2013). Effect of maternal hydration on the amniotic fluid volume during maternal rest in the left lateral decubitus position. *Journal of Ultrasound in Medicine, 32*, 955–961.

Kim, S. Y., Khandelwal, M., Gaughan, J. P., Apgar, M. H., & Reece, E. A. (2003). Is the intrapartum biophysical profile useful? *Obstetrics and Gynecology, 102*(3), 471–476.

Kok, M., Cnossen, J., Gravendeel, L., Van Der Post, J. A., & Mol, B. W. (2009). Ultrasound factors to predict the outcome of external cephalic version: A meta-analysis. *Ultrasound in Obstetrics and Gynecology, 33*, 76–84.

Magann, E. F., Doherty, D. A., Chauhan, S. P., Busch, F. W., Mecacci, F., & Morrison, J. C. (2004). How well do the amniotic fluid index and single deepest pocket indices predict oligohydramnios and hydramnios? *American Journal of Obstetrics and Gynecology, 190*(1), 164–169.

Magann, E. F., Sandlin, A. T., & Ounpraseuth, S. T. (2011). Amniotic fluid volume and the clinical relevance of the sonographically estimated amniotic fluid volume. *Journal of Ultrasound in Medicine, 30*(11), 1573–1585.

Manning, F. A., Baskett, T. F., Morrison, I., & Lange, I. R. (1981). Fetal biophysical scoring: A prospective study in 1,184 high risk patients. *American Journal of Obstetrics and Gynecology, 140*(3), 289–294.

Manning, F. A., Morrison, M. B., Harman, C. R., Lange, I. R., & Menticoglou, S. (1987). Fetal assessment based on fetal biophysical profile scoring: Experience in 19,221 referred high-risk pregnancies. *American Journal of Obstetrics and Gynecology, 157*(4), 880–884.

Mirghani, H. M., Weerasinghe, D. S., Ezimokhai, M., & Smith, J. R. (2003). The effect of maternal fasting on the fetal biophysical profile. *International Journal of Gynaecology and Obstetrics, 81*(1), 17–21.

Morris, J. M., Thompson, K., Smithey, J., Gaffney, G., Cooke, I., Chamberlain, P., . . . MacKenzie, I. Z. (2004). The usefulness of ultrasound assessment of amniotic fluid in predicting adverse outcome in prolonged pregnancy: A prospective blinded observational study. *Obstetrics and Gynecology Survey, 59*(5), 325–326.

Nabhan, A. F., & Abdelmoula, Y. A. (2012). Amniotic fluid index versus single deepest vertical pocket as a screening test for preventing adverse pregnancy outcome. *Journal of Ultrasound in Medicine, 31*(2), 239–244.

Patrelli, T. S., Gizzo, S., Cosmi, E., Carpano, M. G., Di Gangi, S., Pedrazzi, G., . . . Modena, A. B. (2012). Maternal hydration therapy improves the quantity of amniotic fluid and the pregnancy outcome in third-trimester isolated oligohydramnios: A controlled randomized institutional trial. *Journal of Ultrasound in Medicine, 31*, 239.

Phelan, J. P., Ahn, M. O., Smith, C. V., Rutherford, S. E., & Anderson, E. (1987). Amniotic fluid index measurements during pregnancy. *Journal of Reproductive Medicine, 32*(8), 601–604.

Reddy, U., Abuhamad, A., Levine, D., & Saade, G. R. (2014). Fetal imaging: Executive summary of a joint Eunice Kennedy Shriver National Institute of Child Health and Human Development, Society for Maternal-Fetal Medicine, American Institute of Ultrasound in Medicine, American College of Obstetricians and Gynecologists, American College of Radiology, Society for Pediatric Radiology, and Society of Radiologists in Ultrasound Fetal Imaging workshop. *Journal of Ultrasound in Medicine, 33*, 745–757.

Rutherford, S. E., Phelan, J. P., Smith, C. V., & Jacobs, N. (1987). The four quadrant assessment of amniotic fluid volume: An adjunct to antepartum fetal heart rate testing. Part 1. *Obstetrics and Gynecology, 70*(3), 353–356.

Shanks, A., Tuuli, M., Schaecher, C., Odibo, A. O., & Rampersad, R. (2011). Assessing the optimal definition of oligohydramnios associated with adverse neonatal outcomes. *Journal of Ultrasound in Medicine, 30*, 303–307.

Signore, C., Freeman, R., & Sponge, C. (2009). Antenatal testing: A reevaluation. *Obstetrics and Gynecology, 113*(3), 687–701.

Sowmya, K. P., Mudanur, S. R., Padmasri, R., & Lalitha, S. (2017). Modified biophysical profile in antepartum fetal surveillance of high risk pregnancies. *International Journal of Reproduction, Contraception, Obstetrics and Gynecology, 6*(5), 1854–1858.

Vintzileos, A. M., Campbell, W. A., Ingardia, C. J., & Nochimson, D. (1983). The biophysical profile and its predictive value. *Obstetrics and Gynecology, 62*(2), 271–278.

Appendix A

Sample Checklist for Documenting Clinical Proficiency in Ultrasound

Type of Scan	Date Initials	Date Initials	Date Initials	Date Initials	Date Initials	Date Initials	Completed
Chooses correct transducer for type of exam							
Explains procedure to patient							
Adjusts gains							
Utilizes ALARA principle							
Determines fetal presentation							
Fetal cardiac activity							
AFV AFI							
Placental location							
Fetal breathing							
Fetal flexion/extension							
Fetal gross body movement							
Cervical length							
BPD							
HC							

Type of Scan	Date Initials	Date Initials	Date Initials	Date Initials	Date Initials	Date Initials	Completed
Abdominal circumference							
Femur length							
EFW							
EGA							

Note: "Type of Scan" should include any parameter that will be evaluated by the learner and can be specific to what is expected of that learner. The basics of ultrasound physics and instrumentation should be the same for everyone who is going to be using ultrasound.

Supervisor's Signature _____ Date: _____

Learner's Signature _____ Date: _____

Appendix B

Glossary

A

Absorption Decrease in or loss of sound wave penetration due to tissues absorbing the sound waves. The energy is deposited in the medium through which it propagates or moves.

Acoustic enhancement The opposite of attenuation. Sound is not weakened (attenuated) as it passes through a fluid-filled structure; therefore the structure behind it appears to have more echoes than the same tissue beside it.

Acoustic window A structure that has no acoustic impedance (no returning ultrasound signals). This lack of impedance allows for passage of sound and enhanced visualization of deeper structures. The full bladder is an example of an acoustic window.

A-mode ultrasound A single-dimension display consisting of a horizontal baseline, which represents time and or distance with upward (vertical) deflections; spikes indicate the acoustic interfaces.

Anechoic Absence of echoes.

Artifact Distortion of the anatomic structures on the image.

Attenuation Loss of beam amplitude as the sound travels through various tissues; it may be due to absorption, scattering, or reflection.

Axial plane A hypothetical plane parallel to the long axis of an object and along the ultrasound beam's axis. Also referred to as horizontal plane.

Axial resolution The minimum reflector separation along the direction of propagation required to produce separate reflections. The higher the frequency, the better the resolution.

B

Brightness (B) mode A two-dimensional display of ultrasound. The A-mode spikes are electronically converted into dots and displayed at the correct depth from the transducer. Echoes are represented on the display as specific spots that correspond to their point of origin in the body. The brightness of the spot is proportional to the amplitude of the echo.

C

Coronal plane A vertical plane placed at a right angle to a sagittal plane, dividing the body into anterior and posterior portions (right from left). Also called frontal plane. The qualifier "coronal" is used when referring to the view obtained by the probe.

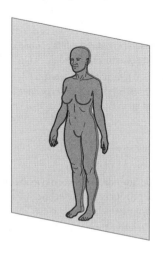

D

Dynamic range A means of adjusting the distance from the transducer as displayed on the image.

E

Echo The returning signal from the interface.
Echogenic A structure that produces echoes.
Echogenicity The relative brightness of returning echoes.

F

Focal position A means of adjusting the region of focus in the image.
Focal zone The region of greatest resolution.

G

Gain A factor that controls the amount of amplification of the returning echoes.

H

Homogeneous Structures that have uniform composition; of uniform appearance and texture.
Hyperechoic A relative term used to describe a structure that has increased brightness of its echoes in comparison to the adjacent structures.
Hypoechoic A relative term used to describe an area that has decreased brightness of its echoes in comparison to the adjacent structures.

I

Interface The boundary between two media (i.e., tissue densities) that produces strong echoes that delineate the boundary of an organ.
Isoechoic A relative term used to describe an area that has an equal distribution of brightness of its echoes.

L

Lateral resolution The ability to separate and define small structures that are perpendicular to the ultrasound beam. It is the minimum reflector separation perpendicular to the direction of propagation required to produce separate reflections. Good lateral resolution is achieved with narrow acoustic beams.
Longitudinal plane A sagittal plane that runs from head to foot and divides the body into right and left halves; it refers to the position of the probe.

M

Median plane The plane created by an imaginary line dividing the body into right and left halves. Also known as the sagittal plane.

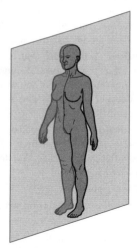

Motion (M) mode A B-mode trace that is moved as a function of time to demonstrate motion. The motion mode displays moving structures along a single line in the ultrasound beam.

P

Pulsed transducer A transducer consisting of one transducer element that functions as both the source and receiving transducers.

R

Reflection Loss of sound waves due to inability to penetrate certain tissues, such as bone.

Resolution The ability to see two different structures as distinct from each other; the parameter of an ultrasound imaging system that characterizes its ability to detect closely spaced interfaces and displays the echoes from those interfaces as distinct and separate objects. The higher the frequency, the better the resolution, and the greater the clarity of the ultrasound image.

Reverberation An artifact that results from a strong echo returning from a large acoustic interface to the transducer. This echo returns to the tissues again, causing additional echoes parallel and equidistant to the first echo.

S

Sagittal plane A plane that runs from head to foot and divides body into right and left halves; used when referring to the view obtained by the probe.

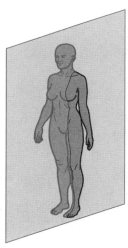

Shadowing Failure of the sound beam to pass through an object. For example, a bone does not allow any sound to pass through it and only shadowing is seen behind it.

Sonolucent Almost devoid of internal echoes or interfaces.

Spectral-flow Doppler A form of ultrasound image display in which the spectrum of flow velocities is represented graphically on the Y-axis and time on the X-axis; both pulsed-wave and continuous-wave Doppler are displayed in this way.

T

Time gain control (TGC) A technique employed to correct varying intensities relative to time traveled, so as to avoid losing information from deeper tissues.

Transverse plane A plane passing through the body at right angles to the sagittal and dorsal planes, and dividing the body into cranial and caudal portions.

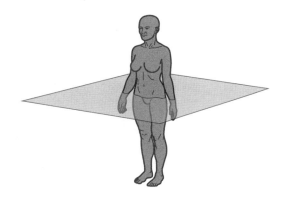

U

Ultrasound Sound with a frequency greater than 2 megahertz or 20,000 hertz (cycles per second). The higher the transducer frequency, the better the resolution, but with loss of penetration.

V

Vertical plane A plane perpendicular to a horizontal plane, dividing the body into left and right, or front and back portions.

Appendix C

Terms for Image Labeling

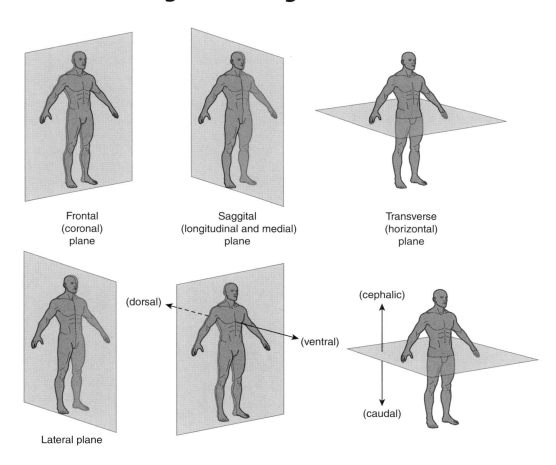

Frontal
(coronal)
plane

Saggital
(longitudinal and medial)
plane

Transverse
(horizontal)
plane

Lateral plane

(dorsal)

(ventral)

(cephalic)

(caudal)

Coronal The long axis of a scan performed from the subject's side, where the slice divides the anterior from the posterior, or the dorsal from the ventral in the long axis.

Transverse A cross-sectional view.

Sagittal (longitudinal) The long axis plane.

Superior, cranial, cephalad, rostral Interchangeable terms indicating the direction toward the head.

Inferior or caudal Indicating the direction toward the feet.

Anterior or ventral A structure lying toward the front of the subject.

Posterior or dorsal A structure ling toward the back of the subject.

Medial Toward the midline.

Lateral Away from the midline.

Proximal Toward the origin.

Distal Away from the origin.

▶ References

American Institute of Ultrasound in Medicine. (2008). *Recommended ultrasound terminology* (3rd ed.). Laurel, MD: Author.

The Free Dictionary by Farlex. (n.d.). Medical dictionary. Retrieved from http://medical-dictionary.thefreedictionary.com

Appendix D

Sample Estimated Fetal Weight Charts

Birthweight percentiles for male singleton live births in Canada, 1986–1988*

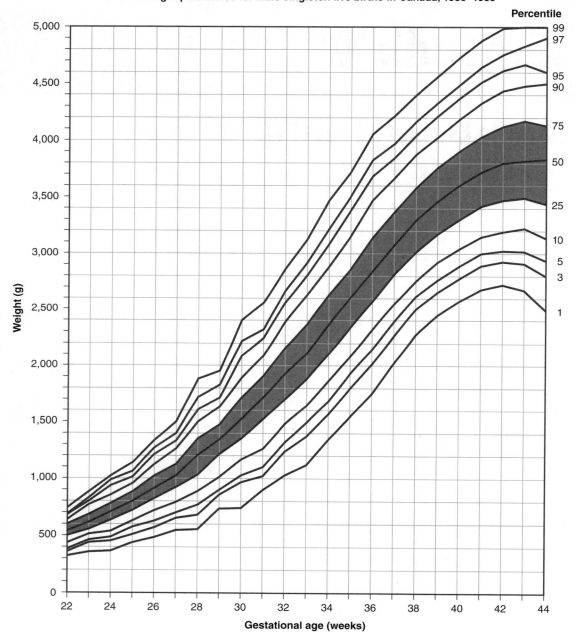

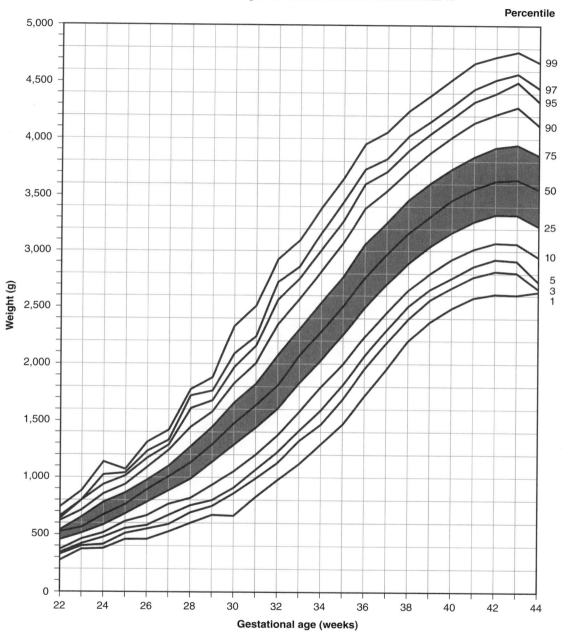

Estimated birth weight for females based in ultrasound EFW

Data from Arbuckle, T. E., Wilkins, R., & Sherman, G. J. (1993). Birthweight percentiles by gestational age in Canada. *Obstetrics and Gynecology, 81*(1), 39–48.

Appendix E

Rationales for Answers to Study Questions

▶ Chapter 1

1. C. A sonologist is a perinatologist or maternal-fetal medicine specialist who has advanced training in fetal ultrasound evaluation.

2. B. Because of the theoretical risk of ultrasound exposure to the fetus, it is recommended that there should be a maternal or fetal indication for ultrasound evaluation.

3. A. A limited ultrasound focuses on a specific area for examination that may be dictated by the clinical situation or indicated based on a finding from a previous ultrasound examination. The limited ultrasound will exclude the majority of the proscribed components of a standard ultrasound.

4. C. A point-of-care ultrasound is generally performed at the bedside to address a specific complaint.

5. B. Determination of ultrasound clinical competency is best confirmed by direct or remote observation by an experienced ultrasound practitioner. However, to lessen ultrasound exposure in pregnant woman, obstetric ultrasound simulators have also been shown to be an alternate method to determine clinical competency.

6. B. During some point-of-care ultrasound examinations performed by nurses based on an AP's or physician's order, it is sufficient to document only that which has been ordered, such as the presenting part or the presence or absence of cardiac activity.

7. C. The utilization of the incorrect transducer for a specific exam will hinder the quality and accuracy of the image, allowing errors in interpretation.

8. B. Because of the theoretical risks of ultrasound exposure to the fetus, the performance of ultrasound examinations in pregnancy should be based on maternal or fetal indications for the exam to acquire specific information.

9. C. When ultrasound images are reviewed retrospectively, an abnormality may be visualized that was missed at the time the ultrasound was performed. The person who performed the first ultrasound failed to perceive that abnormality.

10. B. Whenever a point-of-care or limited ultrasound examination is performed, it is important to explain to the patient that the purpose of the exam is to evaluate a specific organ or system and that it is not a standard ultrasound. For instance, when performing a biophysical profile during pregnancy, it is important to communicate that the exam will not rule out such things as fetal anomalies or placenta previa. It is being done to assess fetal well-being.

▶ Chapter 2

1. B. Acoustic = sound and oscillations = movement back and forth, which is a sound wave with a frequency greater than 20,000 Hz.

2. C. Sound wave frequency is above the range that can be heard by humans, measured as a range above 20,000 Hertz [Hz] or 2 megahertz

[MHz]. Transducers' frequencies are generally defined in terms of MHz)

3. C. Hypoechoic means low echoes returning to the display monitor and will appear dark.

4. B. Propagation is the transmission of sound waves (ultrasound energy) from one place to another. The speed of this transmission is based the type of substance through which energy is moving. For example, the stiffer or denser the matter, the higher the speed.

5. C. Bone is dense and quickly reflects the greatest amount of sound waves back to the transducer.

6. B. It is the transducer that converts electrical energy into mechanical energy within the ultrasonic frequency range.

7. A. The rate at which a vibration occurs per unit of time that constitutes a sound wave. The frequency is determined by each specific transducer.

8. A. Transducer choice is what determines quality of resolution and is based on the frequency of the transducer.

9. B. The higher the frequency, the lower the penetration, and the greater the resolution

10. A. The element oscillates by repeatedly expanding and contracting, generating a sound wave. Each transducer has an inherent frequency that is a function of its crystal composition and shape.

11. C. The propagation speed and the thickness of the piezoelectric element determine the frequency of the transducer. The thinner the element, the higher the frequency.

12. B. The baseline of A-mode represents time or distance with upward deflections that indicate different acoustic interfaces. It is the simplest type of ultrasound. A single transducer scans a line through the body and the returning echoes are plotted on the display screen.

13. A. Sonography in OB/GYN utilizes B-mode or brightness-modulated display in real time. B-mode is two dimensional. The brightness depends upon the amplitude or intensity of the returning echoes.

14. C. M-mode means "motion of an object" that is displayed on a graph allowing for measurement over time. It is a one-dimensional image that is used for analyzing movement within the body, most often in fetal cardiac imaging. It determines amplitude and rate of motion in real time.

15. A. Minimal (but some) return of echoes that produce a darker image with less reflected echoes than surrounding echoes.

16. A. Both continuous wave and pulsed wave measure the direction of the moving blood in relationship to the angle of the transducer beam, which is called Doppler Shift.

17. C. The higher the frequency utilized, the lower the penetration of the sound waves through tissue. So, a high frequency transducer would be used to assess objects closest to the transducer. A lower frequency transducer would be used for visualization of deep structures.

18. A. The transducer range of 3-6 MHz is generally sufficient for most body habitus in OB/GYN imaging, although in women with high BMIs, transabdominal imaging may not be sufficient for interpretable images.

19. C. Longitudinal and transverse are terms used to describe how the transducer is placed on the body of the person being imaged. It is the relationship of the transducer to the body.

20. A. Sagittal and coronal refer to the plane of the actual structure being imaged and shown on the display monitor.

21. B. Because of the way the probe is held as well as introduced into the body, a transverse positioning of the transducer is not possible. Therefore, the only scan planes that can be visualized are longitudinal and coronal.

22. B. With thermal effect, the tissue absorbs the ultrasound wave and heat builds within the tissue, bone having the highest absorption rate of all tissues.

23.   A. Theoretically, cavitation is caused by generation, growth, vibration, and collapse of microbubbles within the tissue. Reducing output power and length of scanning time, as well as the avoidance of color Doppler will reduce the possibility of cavitation.

▸ Chapter 3

1.   A. The bowel will impede the transmission of the sound waves to and through the uterus. The distended bladder lifts the intestines out of the scanning area and provides a fluid-filled acoustic window through which the ultrasound waves will pass.

2.   C. The higher the frequency of the transducer, the higher the resolution, accompanied by a loss of penetration to deeper organs. The transvaginal transducer is placed in close proximity to the organs being visualized and does not require deep penetration of ultrasound waves.

3.   A. The internal iliac vessels are blood filled, thus producing hypoechoic tubular structures in close proximity to the ovaries. Hypoechoic images are generally easier to visualize than hyperechoic structures.

4.   B. There are advantages and limitations to imaging with a full bladder. It does provide an acoustic window in transabdominal ultrasound, but it can displace the position of the uterus in the process, yielding inaccurate results in transvaginal scanning.

5.   A. This myometrial border is composed of longitudinal and circular closely packed smooth-muscle fibers, thus giving the hypoechoic and homogenous (isoechoic) appearance.

6.   C. The endometrium undergoes changes throughout the menstrual cycle, which is then also reflected in the differences in the images.

7.   B. The endometrium changes throughout the menstrual cycle in response to hormone changes. During the follicular phase, estrogen is produced, causing the endometrial lining to grow and thicken to prepare the uterus for pregnancy.

8.   A. This is a set standard so that deviations from normal can be quantified with as much accuracy as possible.

9.   C. It is a good screening test because the evidence has shown a high degree of prediction of normal with a 4 mm or less endometrial stripe.

10.   A. Echoes are only generated from within the cervical canal if there is mucus present in the canal to reflect the soundwaves, which will appear hypogenic.

11.   B. The vaginal walls are tubular, as well as contiguous with each other, producing hypoechoic soundwaves from the tubes, along with stronger signals returning from the center of the tubes.

12.   C. Shadowing appears as a signal void (anechoic) behind structures that strongly absorb or reflect ultrasound waves. It is commonly seen with solid structures, as sound conducts most rapidly in densely packed structures, such as in bone or stones.

13.   C. Fallopian tubes are rarely visualized unless surrounded in intraperitoneal fluid or when thickened or fluid-filled as a result of pelvic inflammatory disease, torsion, ectopic pregnancies, or other pathology.

14.   A. The ovaries are ovoid in appearance. When compared to the myometrium, the ovaries have a lower level of returning echoes (the myometrium will be "brighter") with differing levels of echogenicity throughout (not as "smooth" as the myometrium).

15.   A. Research has shown that follicles can rupture at various sizes, thus making size alone a poor predictor for timing of rupture.

16.   A. Standards have been set for follicular measurement so that there is consistency in data that may be used to prescribe treatments and interventions.

17.   C. The walls can collapse in multiple ways, which will alter the appearance. There may be residual fluid, which will be anechoic or hypoechoic, with the walls' hypoechoic signals of all shapes.

18.   B. As long as IUDs are comprised of plastic, copper, or other solid material, they will be highly reflective of sound waves making them easily distinguishable from surrounding tissue.

19.   B. Whenever a point-of-care or a limited pelvic ultrasound is performed, it is important to consider scheduling a comprehensive or standard pelvic ultrasound to evaluate the remaining anatomy, which will be useful for comparison with future sonograms.

20.   A. Unexpected, inconclusive or positive findings with a point-of-care ultrasound may require immediate consultation. A means of communication with a consultant should be pre-established before adding ultrasound skill to assessment tools to ensure a timely response.

21.   C. Urine is anechoic and easily visualized by ultrasound.

▶ Chapter 4

1.   B. Normal pregnancies can progress even when a double decidual sac sign is not visualized during a first trimester scan. Although the finding is reassuring, its absence in not predictive of an abnormal pregnancy.

2.   A. When fluid is seen within the endometrium, it most likely represents a gestational sac, although the pregnancy may not continue to develop, resulting in an empty sac. Fluid within the endometrium may also represent a pseudogestational sac in the presence of an ectopic pregnancy, but this occurs far less frequently. The vast majority of the time, the fluid represents a gestational sac.

3.   C. Because an intrauterine fluid collection is far more likely to represent a normal pregnancy than anything else, it should be assumed that it is a gestational sac until further evidence proves otherwise to avoid interrupting a normal pregnancy.

4.   C. A first trimester crown–rump measurement is the best estimator of gestational age and establishing an estimated date for delivery.

5.   A. Because the transvaginal transducer allows for earlier embryonic assessment with better visualization, early detection of abnormally progressing pregnancies can occur.

6.   A. Transvaginal sonography allows for early visualization of the gestational sac because of the close proximity of the intrauterine cavity to the transducer.

7.   B. Prior to 14–16 weeks' gestation, the chorion and amnion are visualized as two separate membranes.

8.   C. A normal gestational sac is fluid filled, thus allowing the ultrasound waves to pass through it with few or no returning echoes. It, therefore, appears solid black or nearly solid black and is centrally located within the uterus.

9.   A. Based on early ultrasound research, the normal gestational sac at 4–5 weeks' gestation measured between 2 and 5 mm.

10.   A. Based on the ultrasound literature, the normal gestational sac can be either ellipsoid or circular in shape.

11.   C. The established standard for determining gestational sac size is based on the averaging the three dimensions at the chorionic margin. Using only one or two measurements increases the margin of error.

12.   B. Based on research done on anembryonic pregnancies, it has been clearly determined that by the time the sac measures 25 mm, an embryo should be visible.

13.   A. Based on ultrasound research, it has been determined that an irregularly shaped yolk sac has no predictive value for pregnancy loss.

14.   A. Based on the ultrasound research of normal pregnancies scanned with a transvaginal

transducer, an embryo can be identified as early as 5–6 weeks' gestation.

15. B. Based on ultrasound research of normal pregnancies scanned with a transvaginal transducer, cardiac activity should be visualized when the embryo measures more than 6 mm.

16. C. If no cardiac activity is observed with a transvaginal transducer when the embryo measures greater than 7 mm, a repeat ultrasound should be done in 1 week to ensure a correct diagnosis before determining the pregnancy is nonviable to avoid the possibility of interrupting a normal pregnancy.

17. B. When any assisted reproductive technology is utilized to stimulate oocyte production, multiple gestation may result. To ensure accuracy in counting the number of fetuses, the earliest optimal time has been determined to be between 8 and 10 weeks' gestation.

18. A. Based on ultrasound research, when utilizing a transvaginal transducer, fetal cardiac activity should be visualized by 5 weeks' gestation and/or when the crown–rump length reaches 2–4 mm in 80% of the cases.

19. B. Although Doppler ultrasound can confirm the presence or absence of cardiac activity, the only recommended and safest mode of obtaining that information is with M-mode ultrasound.

20. A. Two ultrasound findings that have the strongest association with fetal loss are a gestational sac size smaller than expected for a specific gestational age and/or a fetal heart rate less than 90–100 bpm. However, neither is a conclusive finding, so a repeat ultrasound 1 week later is recommended to confirm those findings.

21. C. Based on nuchal translucency research, the norms established set the standard for the optimum time to perform these measurements as between 10 and 13 weeks' gestation. Measurements outside these recommendations will have limited, if any, predictive value. These measurements and predictive accuracy do not apply to nuchal *thickening*.

22. A. In order to completely evaluate the adnexa, both a transabdominal and transvaginal scan may be necessary. The TA will provide deeper penetration and better visualization of the deep adnexa, while the TV will provide better resolution of structures closer to the transducer.

23. B. A subchorionic hemorrhage will reflect higher level of echoes than a gestational sac, making it distinguishable from the gestational sac, and it will be located outside of the gestational sac.

24. A. Based on the ultrasound research, in most cases, a subchorionic hemorrhage is not predictive for pregnancy loss, although there is some associated risk of miscarriage and preterm labor.

25. C. Based on ultrasound research, an embryo with a crown–rump length greater than 25 mm with no evidence of cardiac activity is consistent with a fetal demise.

26. A. Based on ultrasound research, a yolk sac should be visualized with a transvaginal transducer once the gestational sac mean diameter reaches 10 mm.

27. C. The incidence of heterotopic pregnancies has increased with the use of ovarian stimulation in assisted reproduction. Under those circumstances in particular, the presence of an intrauterine pregnancy or visualization of a yolk sac does not rule out the possibility of a coexisting ectopic pregnancy.

28. A. In the presence of a positive pregnancy test, an empty uterus may be consistent with an ectopic pregnancy and requires further evaluation.

29. B. Coexisting with an increase in the cesarean birth rate is the increasing incidence of abnormally implanted placentas. An ultrasound finding of placenta previa and low-lying placenta warrants further exploration of the myometrial thickness for a morbidly adherent placenta.

30. B. Based on ultrasound clinical research, an ectopic pregnancy should be considered when the uterus is completely empty in the presence of a ß-hcg greater than 2,000 mIU/mL.

By the time the ß-hcg reaches that level, an intrauterine fluid collection should, at a minimum, be visualized.

▶ Chapter 5

1. C. Standardization of ultrasound parameters established by professional organizations in order to maintain quality of care and safety in ultrasound practice. A point-of-care ultrasound addresses the symptomatology present at the moment of the scan. A standard ultrasound exam in the second trimester includes a specific fetal anatomic survey.

2. C. If a pregnancy has been dated during the first trimester, that date should not be changed based on future ultrasound exams, primarily because of the risk of missing a fetal growth disorder. Pregnancy dating is based on specific fetal anatomic structures, and those structures should show consistent growth throughout the pregnancy.

3. B. Based on standardization of fetal measurement parameters, the fetal biparietal diameter should be obtained utilizing a transverse view.

4. A. Based on standardization of fetal measurement parameters, the thalami should be visualized along with the cavum septum pellucidi to ensure measurements are taken at the correct level.

5. C. When measuring the biparietal diameter, the cursors are place from the outer edge of the fetal skull closest to the transducer to the inner edge of the skull distal to the transducer to ensure accuracy. The returning signals from the distal outer skull may appear thicker due to artifact, which is why it is excluded from the measurement.

6. A. The accuracy of biparietal diameter may be jeopardized by head shape, but the head circumference is not dependent on the head shape. Head shape has no impact on the accuracy of the head circumference.

7. A. Based on ultrasound clinical research, it has been determined that the femur length is most accurate for determining fetal growth from 15–32 weeks' gestation. Femur growth is more variable on either side of that range, and therefore, less reliable.

8. C. The femur is measured in the longitudinal view right along the bone, so the transducer is parallel to femur.

9. C. Based on research, the standardization for measuring the femur includes measurement of the femur diaphysis. Including the epiphysis will yield erroneous results indicating a greater gestational age than is true.

10. C. The epiphyses ossify late in gestation. Prior to 32 weeks' gestation, the epiphysis is less dense so the reflected sound waves are hypoechoic in comparison with the diaphysis which is denser and, therefore, hyperechoic.

11. A. If the distal femur is used as one of the parameters in determining fetal gestational age and weight, it may be inaccurate since the distal femur is subject to posterior artifactual shadowing and may appear bowed in shape.

12. B. Set standardization of fetal anatomic measurement has been established to ensure consistency.

13. C. The fetal abdominal measurements are needed to obtain both fetal age and weight because the abdominal growth provides the best consistency for the calculations.

14. C. Set standardization of fetal anatomic measurements has been established to ensure consistency.

15. A. The abdominal circumference is measured from anterior outer skin edge to posterior outer skin edge because the posterior skin thickness is not impacted by any ultrasound artifacts that are capable of altering bone measurements.

16. B. Research has indicated that fetal growth disorders are more accurately determined if scans are done at a minimum of 3 week intervals to allow for the normal variation in growth rates.

17.   A. Research has shown that the estimated fetal weight predication may be off by 15% in either direction; the estimated weight may be 15% less or 15% greater than the prediction. This rate may be improved when there is consistency in the education and training of the sonographers.

18.   A. The majority of advanced practitioners perform a more limited ultrasound scope of practice than sonographers, and APs generally will not have the education and training to perform fetal anatomic scans. This information should be explained to patients so that there are not unreasonable expectations for the ultrasound results.

19.   C. As a placenta ages, areas of calcification develop and outline the cotyledons. The calcifications are denser than the placenta tissue, and, therefore, reflect brighter sound waves (more hyperechoic than the less hyperechoic placenta).

20.   A. The internal cervical os must be visualized in relationship to the placental edge in order to be accurate in determining the presence or absence of a placenta previa.

21.   C. Contracting myometrium as well as pressure into the uterus from an overly distended bladder can make the tissue appear denser allowing for confusion with actual placental tissue; allowing for the misdiagnosis of a placenta previa.

22.   C. With morbidly adherent placentas, there may be formation of an increasing number of placental lakes. These lakes are hypoechoic or anechoic and, therefore, will appears as "Swiss cheese" or "moth eaten." If placental lakes are seen, a MAP may be present.

23.   A. The sonographic appearance of an abruption varies from the time of fresh bleeding, clotting of that blood, or hematoma formation.

24.   A. A succenturiate placenta has two lobes which can be erroneously identified as two placentas, indicating a twin pregnancy.

25.   C. Placental lakes do reflect some soundwaves, so they are not as anechoic as urine.

26.   A. Based on research, cervical length measurement has the best predictive value when performed after 14 weeks' gestation.

27.   B. Based on research, in most cases both cervical shortening and dilation begin at the internal cervical os and move down to the external os.

28.   C. Based on research, the measurements obtained with the transvaginal transducer are more accurate than those obtained with the abdominal transducer. However, if the abdominal measurements are "long," a follow-up transvaginal scan need not be done.

29.   C. Air bubbles interfere in the transmission of sound waves creating artifactual information and/or an inability to interpret the scan.

30.   B. Based on research, set standardization has been established for consistency in measurement and quality of care. The majority of ultrasound machines do not have the capability of measuring a curvature.

31.   A. The shortest of three cervical length measurements is reported and used for management. This is to ensure that an error in measurement might provide false reassurance.

32.   A. The cervix begins to funnel at the internal os before the cervix begins to dilate. Research has indicated funneling is a predictor of preterm labor and is easily visualized on ultrasound.

33.   B. With funneling present, the cervix is measured from the "bottom" of the funnel to the external os. It will reflect more echoes than the funnel and is the remaining portion of the closed cervix.

▶ Chapter 6

1.   B. Research has shown that fetal tone can be visualized by ultrasound beginning at about 7.5 to 8 weeks' gestation.

2.   C. Research has shown that fetal movement can be visualized by ultrasound by about 8.5-10 weeks' gestation.

3. A. Research has shown that fetal breathing can be visualized by ultrasound by about 20–21 weeks' gestation.

4. A. Research has shown that fetal heart rate accelerations and decelerations become apparent by the end of the second trimester or the beginning of the third trimester.

5. C. Research has shown that chronic deoxygenation of the fetus leads to a loss of fetal heart rate accelerations and decelerations, loss of breathing movements, loss of tone, and decreased amniotic fluid, in that order. Factors other than chronic deoxygenation may cause a loss of an individual parameter; but in the presence of chronic deoxygenation, the order of the above losses appears to hold true.

6. B. Chronic oxygen deprivation causes the fetus to shunt blood away from nonvital organs to the vital organs. This diminishment of blood flow to the kidneys causes decreased urine output, which is the primary substance in amniotic fluid.

7. B. The standardization is based on research showing the designated fetal behaviors in the biophysical profile had the highest predictability for a good outcome. The criteria remain as established.

8. C. The standardization is based on research showing the designated fetal behaviors in the biophysical profile had the highest predictability for a good outcome. The criteria remain as established.

9. B. The standardization is based on research showing the designated fetal behaviors in the biophysical profile had the highest predictability for a good outcome. The criteria remain as established.

10. C. Clinical research has established that oligohydramnios be defined as a less than 2-cm vertical pocket of amniotic fluid, as utilization of other methods may lead to more interventions for oligohydramnios.

11. A. Research has shown that Doppler flow assessment of amniotic fluid has a high false-positive rate in the diagnosis of oligohydramnios.

12. C. The fetal diaphragm is one of the best landmarks to use when assessing fetal breathing movements. The diaphragm is easily located by ultrasound.

Appendix F

Additional Resources

Ultrasound certification (American Registry for Diagnostic Medical Sonography): www.ardms.org

Society for Diagnostic Medical Sonography: www.sdms.org

American Institute of Ultrasound in Medicine: www.aium.org

Cervical length measurement certification (Cervical Length Education and Review [CLEAR]): https://clear.perinatalquality.org

Index

Note: Page numbers followed by *b*, *f* and *t* indicate boxes, figures and tables respectively.